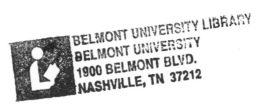

The Pelvic Girdle

To Cliff Fowler and the memory of David Lamb

For Churchill Livingstone

Editorial Director, Health Sciences: Mary Law
Project Manager: Ewan Halley / Valerie Burgess
Project Editor: Dinah Thom
Design Direction: Judith Wright
Indexer: Nina Boyd

The Pelvic Girdle

An approach to the examination and treatment of the lumbo-pelvic-hip region

Diane Lee BSR MCPA FCAMP
Instructor/Examiner for the Orthopaedic Division of the Canadian Physiotherapy Association

Foreword by

Andry Vleeming PhD
Director, Spine and Joint Centre, Rotterdam, and Head of the Musculoskeletal System Research Group,
Department of Anatomy, Faculty of Medicine and Health Sciences, Erasmus University,
Rotterdam, The Netherlands

SECOND EDITION

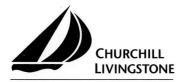

CHURCHILL LIVINGSTONE

EDINBURGH LONDON NEW YORK PHILADELPHIA SYDNEY TORONTO 1999

CHURCHILL LIVINGSTONE
An imprint of Harcourt Brace and Company Limited

Churchill Livingstone, Robert Stevenson House, 1–3
Baxter's Place, Leith Walk, Edinburgh EH1 3AF, UK

First Edition 1989
Second Edition 1999

ISBN 0443 05814 8

British Library of Cataloguing in Publication Data
A catalogue record for this book is available from the British
Library.

Library of Congress Cataloging in Publication Data
A catalogue record for this book is available from the
Library of Congress.

Medical knowledge is constantly changing. As new
information becomes available, changes in treatment,
procedures, equipment and the use of drugs become
necessary. The author and the publishers have, as far as it is
possible, taken care to ensure that the information given in
this text is accurate and up to date. However, readers are
strongly advised to confirm that the information, especially
with regard to drug usage, complies with current legislation
and standards of practice.

The
publisher's
policy is to use
paper manufactured
from sustainable forests

Printed in China
CTPS/01

Contents

Foreword

For decades, interest in both the anatomy and the biomechanics of the pelvis has been minimal. This is an understandable reaction to the enthusiasm at the beginning of this century, when many believed that most lumbopelvic problems were exclusively the result of malfunctions of the sacroiliac joint. The model of the herniated disc was more reassuring in that there appeared to be a relationship between an anatomical impairment and clinical consequences. Unfortunately, this model was disproportionately used to explain how pain experienced in the pelvis originated mainly from impairments in the lumbar spine, and that pain in the pelvis was nothing more than radiating pain.

During this time, many patients, in agony with severe pelvic pain, were not believed because no anatomical impairment could be found to explain their symptoms. The basic theory of how load is transferred between the spine, pelvis and legs was not available, and consequently there was no understanding of how pathomechanics could lead to lumbopelvic pain. From a biomechanical and anatomical point of view, it is amazing how the pelvis was overlooked for so many years in the attempt to understand the structure and function of the musculoskeletal system.

Overlooking the pelvis could be due to the questions being asked. Anatomical models that divide the body into separate parts were thought sufficient to answer the questions. Specific structures were sought which when disrupted could explain the prevalence of lumbopelvic pain in our society. For the main part of this century, research has focused on where the pain is located and how it relates to impaired structures (anatomical model). The tendency to search for quantifiable 'physical' impairments within isolated structures prevailed. When the faulty structure was identified, predominantly single modality treatment was used to solve the problem. If this approach failed, patients were classified as having a psychosomatic problem.

The practical consequence of this approach has been that complex interactive kinematic systems were analysed and treated as isolated parts with the use of increasingly sophisticated technology. This approach neglects the structure and function of the kinematic system as a whole. Subsequently, treatment of pelvic pain and dysfunction became divided amongst several specialties, each dealing with different parts of the anatomy!

As knowledge of *functional* anatomy, physiology, biomechanics and neurology emerged, the questions changed. We now realize that understanding musculoskeletal problems requires knowledge of how loads are transferred through the body and how deficiencies in one part can influence the function of the entire system. With these questions in mind, it becomes of paramount importance to understand the function of the pelvis. Using a simple model of three levers (two legs and the spine) acting on the pelvis (basic bony platform), it is not difficult to perceive that this platform, which is capable of extrinsic and intrinsic motion, must be stabilized before levers (spine and legs) can act on it. A model of biomechanical function leads to biomechanical treatments, a great emotional relief for patients shattered by chronic pelvic pain.

Diane Lee is one of the first clinicians to fathom the importance of a more conscientious study of the pelvis. Patients with severe and incomprehensible pelvic problems were sent to her clinic, often as a last attempt to cure those believed to have mainly unrealistic complaints. To become more effective in the treatment of these patients, Diane Lee strove to rapidly incorporate and apply the latest fundamental and clinical data. When she presented her work during the First Interdisciplinary World Congress on Low Back Pain she had managed to incorporate in her presentation most of the relevant data of speakers at that same conference.

It is a pleasure to write this foreword for a book which I sincerely believe delivers a true state-of-the-art text to those clinicians and other interested people who consider effective treatment of pelvic problems essential in their practices. I also believe that this book is written by one of the most original clinicians working in the field of the musculoskeletal system. With the appearance of the second edition, it becomes obvious how fast our knowledge of the pelvis is developing. I am convinced that this book will bring the latest, valuable knowledge to all readers.

1998   Andry Vleeming

Preface to the Second Edition

There have been many exciting advances in the understanding of the lumbo-pelvic-hip region over the last decade, some of which have led to significant changes in both assessment and treatment. While controversy still exists over the reliability and specificity of manual diagnostic procedures, certainty prevails in other areas. Over the last decade, my work has been significantly influenced by others, namely the research teams from Erasmus University in Rotterdam and the University of Queensland in Brisbane. In particular, the work of Dr Andry Vleeming and Dr Chris Snijders (from the Erasmus team) on the functional biomechanical model of the lumbar spine, pelvis and lower extremity has led to significant changes in how load is thought to be transferred from the trunk to the lower extremity. In addition, the research of Dr Paul Hodges, Dr Julie Hides, Dr Carolyn Richardson and Gwendolyn Jull (from the University of Queensland team) on the function of the inner unit of muscles, and their evidence-based principles of exercise training, have formed the foundation for the stabilization program presented in this text.

My particular contribution over the past ten years has been to describe specific mobility and stability assessment techniques (joint play) which are used clinically to determine the status of mobility of the sacroiliac joint. I am indebted to Dr Andry Vleeming for the hours of discussion which have led to the 'new model' of impaired load transfer through joints. In this new model, joint play tests are essential for understanding the abnormal movements which can occur in a normal neutral zone. This work is yet to be published and is presented here with his permission.

Once again, I would like to extend my gratitude to Mr Frank Crymble who is responsible for all the line drawings and clinical photographs in this text; some are from the first edition while many are new. I would also like to express my thanks to Dr Frank Willard for permitting me to reproduce in Chapter 4 his excellent photographs of the anatomical dissections.

The photograph on the cover of this edition was taken by a colleague, Evan Zaleschuk, while travelling in India. I am grateful to him for allowing me to share it with you. The stone arch reflects the stability role of the pelvic girdle while the bicycle represents mobility. The open gate reminds us to keep an open mind when presented with a different view of a common problem.

Finally, words are hard to find which express my appreciation for my colleagues at work, whose support is truly remarkable, and for my family, who have endured once again the endless hours a task such as this demands.

1998   Diane Lee

Preface to the First Edition

In 1980 it was my good fortune to have the opportunity to study with one of the leaders in manipulative therapy, Mr Cliff Fowler. Over the ensuing years I was shown how to treat people, not conditions, how to integrate academic knowledge with clinical experience and how to learn from every patient's story. At that time every story seemed to have a different stage, different players and a different plot. Through the consistent use of a basic subjective and objective examination it became apparent that there were common patterns of lumbo-pelvic-hip dysfunction. From this, a logical approach to treatment has evolved.

The intent of this text is to assist the clinician in the development of a logical approach to the examination and treatment of the lumbo-pelvic-hip region based on the known anatomy, physiology and biomechanics.

Chapter 1 is a historical review of the trends of thought from Hippocrates to the present day with respect to the function and dysfunction of the pelvic girdle. Chapter 2 outlines the evolution and comparative anatomy of the pelvis, followed by a description of the anatomical changes which have occurred as a result of bipedalism. This chapter is co-authored by Mr Jim Meadows whom I would like to thank, both for this contribution and for the many hours of stimulating and thought-provoking discussions.

The embryology, development and aging of the pelvic girdle is described and illustrated in Chapter 3. I would like to express my thanks to Dr J. M. Walker for providing the original photographs which illustrate the cavitation of the sacroiliac joint in the fetus, the variability in the depth of the cartilage lining the articular surfaces, and the subsequent erosion and fibrous intra-articular fusion which occurs with age. The differences between the articular cartilage lining the ilium and the sacrum, as well as the changes associated with advancing age, are clearly illustrated in the original color photographs kindly provided by Dr J. D. Cassidy, to whom I would like to extend my gratitude.

Chapter 4 describes and illustrates the osteology, arthrology, myology, neurology and angiology of the lumbo-pelvic-hip complex pertinent to the description and evaluation of the biomechanics of the region, which is given in Chapter 5. The theoretical section of this text is completed (Ch. 6) with a brief description of the three phases of wound repair. The clinical application of this healing process is applied in the subsequent treatment sections of Chapters 8, 9 and 10.

Chapter 7 describes and illustrates the basic subjective and objective examination of the lumbo-pelvic-hip complex. The following three chapters describe and illustrate the evaluation and treatment of the common clinical syndromes seen at the lumbosacral junction, the pelvic girdle and the hip. The text is concluded with a description of the myofascial, postural and ergonomic components of therapy.

As research expands and clarifies our knowledge of the biomechanics of this region, the examination and treatment techniques can become more specific. It is hoped that this work will stimulate further research into the integrated function of the lumbar spine, the pelvic girdle and the hip, and simultaneously facilitate treatment.

I would like to extend my thanks and recognition to Mr Frank Crymble who was responsible for all the line drawings and photographs in this text. His untiring attention to detail, as well as his anatomical and artistic expertise, made working with him a pleasure. I would also like to express my appreciation and gratitude to my colleagues Mari Walsh, Jim Meadows, Cliff Fowler and Erl Pettman for their constructive reviews of this text in progress and for keeping me focused on the task at hand. Finally, to Thomas, Michael and Chelsea, for all of the hours endured, thank you.

1989   Diane Lee

Glossary of terms

Kinematics	the study of movement
Kinetics	the study of forces
Osteo-	bone
Arthro-	joint
Myo-	muscle
Osteokinematics	the study of motion of bones regardless of the motion of the joints
Arthrokinematics	the study of motion of joints regardless of the motion of the bones
Myokinematics	the study of motion of bones produced by the contraction of the muscle
Osteokinetics	the study of forces met by the bones
Arthrokinetics	the study of forces met by the joints
Myokinetics	the study of forces met by the muscles

1

Introduction: historical review

The first medical practitioners to record interest in the pelvic girdle were the obstetricians of Hippocrates' era. Hippocrates (460–377 BC) and Vesalius (AD 1543) felt that under normal conditions the sacroiliac joints were immobile; however, others (Paré 1643) felt that motion was apparent during pregnancy (Weisl 1955). This view was upheld until De Diemerbroeck (1689) demonstrated that mobility of the sacroiliac joint could occur apart from pregnancy. From the 17th century until recently, a controversy has existed as to the classification and composition of the sacroiliac joint, the quantity, if any, of motion, and the specific biomechanics which accompany movement of the lower extremities and the trunk.

The joint has been implicated as the cause of many symptoms including sciatica; in fact, at the turn of this century Albee and Goldthwait & Osgood (Albee 1909, Goldthwait & Osgood 1905) proposed that sciatica developed from direct pressure on the lumbosacral plexus as it crossed the anterior aspect of the sacroiliac joint. This pressure was thought to be caused by 'subluxed, relaxed or diseased sacroiliac joints' (Meisenbach 1911). Treatment consisted of manipulative reduction of the sacrum followed by immobilization, in plaster, in spinal hyperextension for six months. Following the classic paper by Mixter & Barr (1934) on prolapsed intervertebral discs and the clinical ramifications of pressure on the lumbosacral nerve roots intra-spinally, the sacroiliac joint was felt to be less significant and lesions of this articulation were regarded as rare (Cyriax 1954).

Research over the last 50 years has revealed significant information pertaining to the anatomy and function of the pelvic girdle. In 1992, the first interdisciplinary world congress on low back pain and its relation to the sacroiliac joint (Vleeming et al 1992a) exposed the current state of knowledge in this area and a challenge was put forth at that time to apply some scientific research to the topic. Three years later, the second world congress (Vleeming et al 1995b) brought forth a wealth of exceptional information which has become part of the foundation for rehabilitation of instability within the pelvic girdle.

The anatomy and integrated function of the low back, pelvic girdle and lower extremity is more clearly understood. The clinical evaluation procedures and treatment measures are still subjects open to debate and research. Once again, it is appropriate to record the current thoughts on the anatomy, biomechanics, and clinical syndromes of the lumbo-pelvic-hip complex. The model is clearer, and consistent with the research findings. The examination and treatment techniques are more specific and follow the biomechanical model. Further research to establish the reliability and validity of these methods is still necessary.

2

Evolution and comparative anatomy

In collaboration with

James Meadows MCPA MCSP FCAMT

Instructor for the Orthopaedic Division of the Canadian Physiotherapy Association and the North American Institute of Orthopaedic Manipulative Therapy. Founder and director of Swodeam Consulting.

Author's note. The evolution of bipedalism and the consequential anatomical changes which have occurred provide some insight into the structure and function of the lumbo-pelvic-hip complex of Homo sapiens. For this contribution, I am indebted to Jim Meadows for his many hours of research into this subject.

INTRODUCTION

The human lumbo-pelvic-hip region, while in many respects unique in the animal world for its evolutionary adaptation to orthograde bipedalism, is based on a design originating almost half a billion years ago. The absence of fossils of human pelves older than five million years supports the assumption that the adaptation to bipedalism is recent. This chapter will briefly outline the evolutionary steps which have facilitated man's gait. Subsequently, the changes in man's structure and posture as a result of bipedalism will be described.

EVOLUTION OF THE PELVIC GIRDLE

The pelvic girdle first appeared (Encyclopedia Britannica 1981, Gracovetsky & Farfan 1986, Nelson & Jurnaim 1985, Romer 1959, Stein & Rowe 1982, Young 1981) as a pair of small cartilaginous elements lying in the abdomen of the primitive fish. The 'fin fold' theory maintains that lateral folds formed in the ancient fish to prevent rolling and buckling of the undulating body. As the folds contributed to propulsion and steering, they gradually began to fragment. From this fragmentation, two paired lateral fins were formed, the pectoral and pelvic fins. The pectoral fin was the primary propeller and was the largest and the most stable of the two. Since stability was not a functional requirement of the pelvic girdle, there was no need for axial attachment nor attachment between the two sides.

With migration onto land, the pelvic fin rapidly developed into the powerhouse of locomotion and consequently increased stability of the pelvic girdle was required. The pectoral fin (and its later development the forelimb), was relegated to the role of steering—a reversal of the original roles.

Stabilization of the pelvic girdle

The pelvic girdle has evolved towards increased stability both at the pubic symphysis and at the sacroiliac joints. The original innominate bone contained two elements which together formed the puboischium. During the stabilization process, the puboischium enlarged and united with the opposite side via the puboischial symphysis. Intra-pelvic stability was subsequently increased; however, stability between the primitive innominate bone and the axial skeleton was also required. A dorsal projection developed on the puboischium (ultimately forming the ilium) directed towards the axial skeleton.

Simultaneously, the costal element of the axial skeleton enlarged and fused with one (or more) pre-anal vertebra to form the sacrum. The iliac projection of the primitive innominate bone and the enlarged costal process of the primitive sacrum formed the first sacroiliac joint. The initial union was ligamentous. Thus, direct articulation between the axial and appendicular skeletons occurred. At this stage, the pelvic girdle had a full inventory of the elements that are present today in all tetrapods.

The number of vertebrae which contribute to the sacrum varies from species to species and depends on the degree of stability or mobility required at the sacroiliac joint. Many amphibians

and reptiles have only one or two sacral vertebrae whereas higher mammals have five. The extreme of sacral development is found in the bird where the synsacrum includes the fusion of the sacral, lumbar and caudal thoracic vertebrae. This, together with the huge sternum, provides the stability necessary for anchoring the muscles which move the wings.

As the locomotive pattern of the vertebrates progressed from crawling to the linear-limb quadripedal and bipedal gait of the advanced mammals, the role of the ilium became more significant. The bone provided the major pelvic attachment for the limb musculature as well as the articular surface for the sacroiliac joint.

COMPARATIVE ANATOMY

The structure of man's pelvic girdle reflects the adaptation required for bipedal gait (Basmajian & Deluca 1985, Farfan 1978, Goodall 1979, Keagy & Brumlik 1966, Nelson & Jurmain 1985, Rodman & McHenry 1980, Stein & Rowe 1982, Swindler & Wood 1982, Tuttle 1975, Warwick & Williams 1989) (Fig. 2.1). The surface area of the ilia has increased whereas the length of the ischium and the pubis has decreased. The posterior muscles have lost some bulk secondary to the increased stability of the sacroiliac joint. Sufficient mobility of the sacroiliac joint has been maintained for bipedalism.

Sacrum

The sacrum has increased in size thus accommodating the increased osseous attachment of the gluteus maximus muscle. The articular surface of the sacroiliac joint has also increased in size and facilitates the increased compression produced in bipedal stance. The surface itself has become more incongruous (Ch. 3) and facilitates intra-pelvic stability.

Innominate

The ilia have undergone dramatic changes in response to bipedalism. The bone has twisted

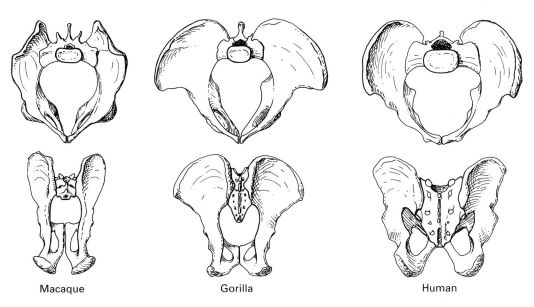

Macaque   Gorilla   Human

Figure 2.1 Comparative anatomy of the pelvic girdle. (Redrawn from Stein & Rowe 1982.)

(Fig. 2.1) such that the lateral aspect is now directed anteriorly. The gluteus medius and minimus muscles have migrated anteriorly and their function has subsequently changed. In the ape, the gluteus medius and minimus muscles are femoral extensors, while in man they act as femoral abductors (Fig. 2.2) and thus prevent a Trendelenburg gait.

In addition to the reorientation of the ilium, a fossa has developed (the iliac fossa) which increases the surface area available for the attachment of the gluteal and iliacus muscles. The reduction in extensor power caused by the anterior migration of the gluteus medius and minimus muscles is therefore compensated for. The iliac fossa also facilitates the enlargement of the iliacus muscle which plays a significant role in the maintenance of man's erect posture.

The anatomical changes apparent in the ischium reflect the alteration in function of the hamstring muscle group (see below). Although these muscles have continued to be involved in femoral extension, constant activity is not a requirement of bipedal stance in man. Subsequently, the ischial body and tuberosity have become reduced in both length and width (Fig. 2.1). The vertical dimension of the pubic

symphysis has also decreased with the evolution of efficient bipedal gait.

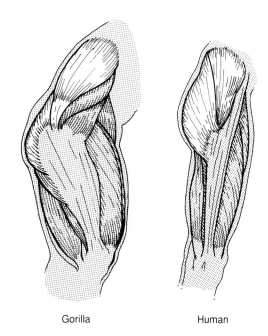

Gorilla   Human

Figure 2.2 The gluteus medius and minimus muscles in the gorilla function as femoral extensors while in man they act as femoral abductors.

3

Embryology, development and aging

EMBRYOLOGY AND DEVELOPMENT

Development of bones

Sacrum

The sacrum derives its name from the Latin word *sacer* meaning sacred. It is thought that the sacrum was the only bone to be preserved following the burning of a witch and as such must have been sacred. Fryette credits the 'ancient Phallic Worshipers [for naming] the base of the spine the Sacred Bone' (Fryette 1954).

The bone is derived from the fusion of five mesodermal somites. During the 4th embryonic week, 42 to 44 pairs of somites arise from the paraxial mesoderm. Although not consistently, the sacrum evolves from the 31st to the 35th somites each of which divides into three components—the sclerotome, myotome and dermatome (Fig. 3.1). The sclerotome multiplies and migrates both ventrally and dorsally to surround the notochord and the evolving spinal cord. Subsequently, each sclerotome divides into equal cranial and caudal components separated by a sclerotomic fissure which in the sacrum progresses to develop a rudimentary intervertebral disc composed of fibrocartilage. The adjacent sclerotomic segments then fuse to form the centrum of the sacral vertebral body. The dorsal aspect of the sclerotome, which has migrated posteriorly, forms the vertebral arch (the neural arch is part of this), while the ventrolateral aspect becomes the costal process (ala of the sacrum) (Fig. 3.2). This process

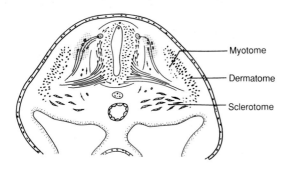

Figure 3.1 Differentiation of the mesodermal somite into sclerotome, myotome and dermatome. (Redrawn from Warwick & Williams 1989.)

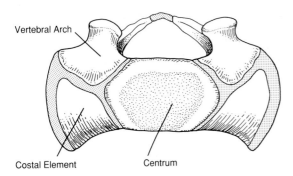

Figure 3.2 The sclerotome of the future sacrum differentiates into three parts—the centrum, the vertebral arch and the costal element or process.

appears only in the upper two or three sacral segments and is responsible for forming the auricular sacral surface.

Chondrification of the sacrum precedes ossification and begins during the 6th embryonic week (Rothman & Simeone 1975). The primary ossification centers for the centrum and each half of the vertebral arch appear between the 10th and the 20th week, while the primary centers for the costal elements appear later, between the 6th and the 8th month.

The three components of the sacral segment (Fig. 3.2), the costal element, the vertebral arch and the centrum, remain separated by hyaline cartilage up until 2 to 5 years of age when the costal element (ala of the sacrum) unites with the vertebral arch. This unit then fuses to the centrum and to the other vertebral arch in the 8th year.

The conjoined costal element, vertebral arch and centrum of each sacral segment remain separated from those above and below by hyaline cartilage laterally and by fibrocartilage medially (Fig. 3.3). A cartilaginous epiphysis extends the entire length of the lateral aspect of the sacrum. Fusion of the sacral segments occurs after puberty in a caudocranial direction with the simultaneous appearance of secondary ossification centers for the centrum, spinous process, transverse processes and costal elements. The adjacent margins of the sacral vertebrae ossify after the 20th year; however, the central portion of the intervertebral disc can remain unossified even after middle life.

Innominate

The innominate has a Latin derivation *innominatus*, meaning having no name. It appears during the 7th embryonic week as three bones, the ilium, the ischium and the pubis, which are derived from a small proliferating mass of mesenchyme from the somatopleure in the developing limb bud. Three primary ossification centers appear before birth, one for the ilium above the sciatic notch during the 8th intrauterine week, one for the ischium in the body of the bone during the 4th month and one for the pubis in the superior ramus between the 4th and 5th months. At birth, the iliac crest, the acetabular fossa and the inferior ischiopubic ramus are cartilaginous (Fig. 3.4). The latter ossifies during the 7th to 8th year. The iliac crest and the acetabular fossa develop secondary ossification centers during puberty but can remain unossified until 25 years of age.

When treating adolescents, it is pertinent to recall the stage of development before applying vigorous mobilization or manipulation techniques.

Development of joints

Sacroiliac joint

According to Bellamy et al (1983), the development of the sacroiliac joint commences during

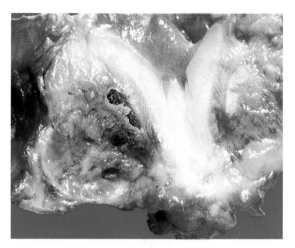

Plate 1   Sacroiliac joint of a fetus at 37 weeks of gestation. Note that the fibrocartilage lining the articular surface of the ilium is bluer than the hyaline cartilage lining the articular surface of the sacrum.

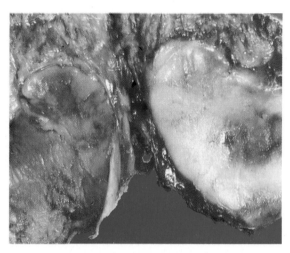

Plate 3   Sacroiliac joint of a male, 17 years of age (the sacral surface is on the right). Note the dull, rough fibrocartilage lining the articular surface of the ilium.

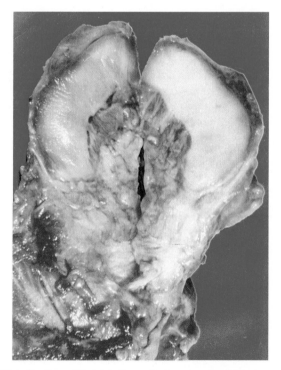

Plate 2   Sacroiliac joint of a male, 3 years of age (the sacral surface is on the right). Note the blue, dull fibrocartilage lining the articular surface of the ilium.

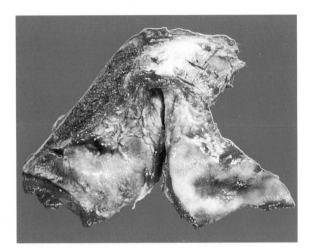

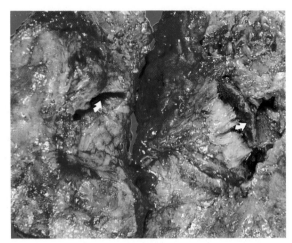

Plate 4 Sacroiliac joint of a male, 40 years of age (the sacral surface is on the right).

Plate 5 Sacroiliac joint of a female, 72 years of age (the sacral surface is on the left). Note the marked loss of articular cartilage on both sides of the joint as well as the presence of an accessory sacroiliac joint (arrows). (Plates 1–5 are reproduced from Bowen & Cassidy 1981 with permission of the publishers Harper and Rowe.)

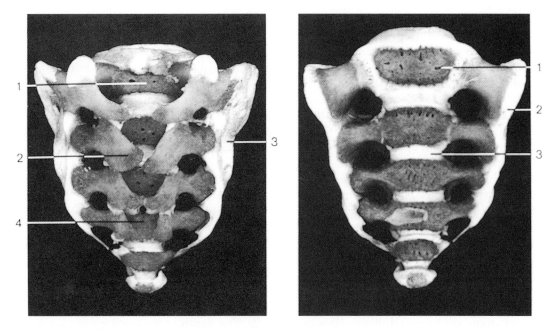

Figure 3.3 Ossification of the sacrum. *Left*—Posterior aspect: note the centrum (1), the vertebral arch (2), the lateral epiphysis (3) and the sacral canal (4). *Right*—Anterior aspect: note the centrum (1), the lateral epiphysis (2) and the intervertebral disc (3). (Reproduced with permission from Rohen & Yokochi 1983.)

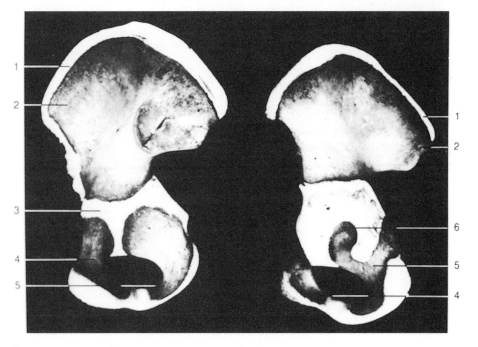

Figure 3.4 Ossification of the innominate. Note the cartilage of the iliac crest (1), the ilium (2), the cartilage separating the ilium, pubis and ischium (3), the pubis (4), the ischium (5) and the acetabulum (6). (Reproduced with permission from Rohen & Yokochi 1983.)

the 8th week of intrauterine life. As in other synovial joints, a trilayer structure initially appears in the mesenchyme between the ilium and the costal element of the sacrum. Cavitation begins both peripherally and centrally by the 10th week and by the 13th week the enlarged cavities are separated by fibrous septae. These findings are not consistent with Walker's (1984, 1986) study of 36 fetuses in which she noted that cavitation did not begin until the 32nd week (Fig. 3.5). The stage at which cavitation is complete and the fibrous bands disappear is controversial. Bellamy et al (1983) state that the cavity is fully developed by the 8th month and that the fibrous septae soon disappear whilst Walker (1986) notes that unlike most synovial joints which show complete cavitation by the 12th week, the sacroiliac joint remains separated by fibrous bands at birth and she questions their persistence in some joints into adulthood. Bowen & Cassidy (1981) report that the 10 specimens

studied in this age group did not contain the fibrous septae previously noted in late fetal life. Schunke (1938) was the first to describe these intra-articular bands and felt that they disappeared in the first year of life.

The synovium of the joint develops from the mesenchyme at the edges of the primordial cavity, as does the articular capsule which is thin and pliable at this stage (Bowen & Cassidy 1981). All investigators note (Bowen & Cassidy 1981, Schunke 1938, Walker 1986) the macroscopic and microscopic differences between the cartilage which lines the articular surfaces of the ilium and the sacrum, although the specific histological components of these surfaces remain a controversial issue.

The ilium is lined with a type of fibrocartilage which is bluer, duller and more striated than the hyaline cartilage which lines the sacrum (Plates 1, 2). The depth of the cartilage is also different. According to Bowen & Cassidy (1981), the sacral

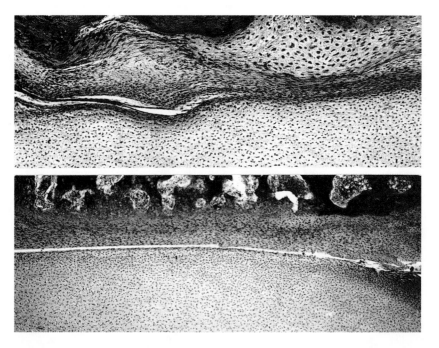

Figure 3.5 Cavitation of the sacroiliac joint. *Top*—Sacroiliac joint of a fetus at 16 weeks of gestation. Note the proximity of the iliac bone to the joint surface, the partial cavitation of the joint and the presence of a fibrous band connecting the two surfaces. *Bottom*— Sacroiliac joint of a fetus at 34 weeks of gestation. Note that cavitation is almost complete except for a few loose fibrous bands. (Reproduced with permission from Walker 1986.)

hyaline cartilage is 3 to 5 times thicker than the iliac fibrocartilage. This is consistent with the findings of Schunke (1938) and MacDonald & Hunt (1951), but differs from the studies of Walker (1986) who found that the sacral hyaline cartilage was 1.7 times thicker than the iliac fibrocartilage, although this finding may vary depending upon which aspect of the joint was being studied. All agree that the corresponding articular surfaces were smooth and flat at this stage, although Walker (1984) found elevations and depressions on her full-term infants as well. Bowen & Cassidy (1981) note that during handling of the fetal pelves, the joint was capable of gliding in a multitude of directions.

Pubic symphysis and hip joint

Very few investigators have researched the developmental anatomy of the pubic symphysis and a reference could not be found pertaining to the anatomical changes which may occur at this articulation with advancing age.

It is beyond the scope of this text to describe the detailed embryology of the hip joint; however, several references are included for the interested reader (Siffert & Feldman 1980, Strayer 1971, Walker 1980a, 1980b, 1981, Watanabe 1974).

THE SACROILIAC JOINT AND AGING

At birth, the pelvic girdle is far from complete developmentally. A major part of the unit is cartilaginous and the articular anatomy contributes little to intra-pelvic stability. The changes which occur within the sacroiliac joints over the next seven decades are significant for the biomechanics, assessment and treatment of the pelvic girdle in the varying age groups.

The first decade (0–10 years)

Bowen & Cassidy (1981) studied seven pelves in this age group and report that the surfaces of the sacroiliac joint remain primarily flat (Plate 2) with the major restraint to passive motion being provided by the very strong interosseous liga-

ments. The articular cartilage remains as noted prenatally.

The second and third decades (11–30 years)

The availability of cadavers for investigation in this age group is limited; the data obtained are, therefore, based on few specimens. Sashin's (1930) investigation of age-related intra-articular changes is perhaps the most extensive; 42 specimens in his study belonged to this age group. The study of Resnick et al (1975) included only two specimens, MacDonald & Hunt's (1951) seven, Bowen & Cassidy's (1981) seven, and Walker's (1986) none.

Early in the second decade the sacroiliac joint appears planar; however, by the beginning of the third decade all specimens manifest a convex ridge which runs along the entire length of the articular surface of the ilium apposed to a corresponding sacral groove (Bowen & Cassidy 1981, Vleeming et al 1990a) (Fig. 3.6). The iliac fibrocartilaginous surface is duller, rougher and intermittently coated with fibrous plaques (Plate 3). The deep articular cartilage is microscopically normal, but the superficial layers are fibrillated and some crevice formation and erosion occurs by the end of the third decade. The sacral hyaline cartilage takes on a yellowish hue although macroscopic changes are not evident at this stage. The collagen content of the fibrous capsule increases, thus reducing its extensibility. Passive articular motion is limited to a small angular motion coupled with a few millimetres of translation (Ch. 5).

The fourth and fifth decades (31–50 years)

Several investigators (Bowen & Cassidy 1981, Schunke 1938, Walker 1984, 1986) feel that the changes noted in the articular surfaces during this stage represent a degenerative process. The changes occur earlier in males (fourth decade) than females (fifth decade). Vleeming et al (1990a,b) feel that since these changes are

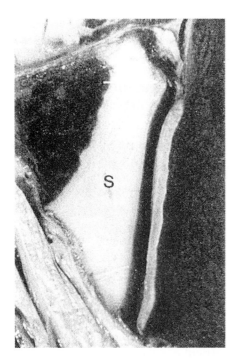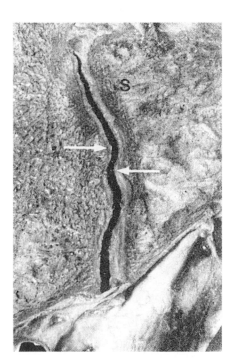

Figure 3.6 A coronal section through two embalmed male specimens, the left aged 12 years and the right over 60 years. Note the planar nature of the sacroiliac joint in the young (S denotes the sacrum) and the presence of ridges and grooves (arrows) in the old. (Reproduced with permission from Vleeming et al 1990a.)

asymptomatic in most, they reflect a functional adaptation secondary to an increase in body weight during puberty and not a degenerative process. They studied the effects of the cartilage texture on the friction coefficient of the joint (Vleeming et al 1990b) and found that together with the development of ridges and grooves, the fibrillated surface increased friction and thus stability of the sacroiliac joint. This was felt to reflect an adaptation to bipedalism.

The articular surfaces increase in irregularity with marked fibrillation occurring on the iliac side by the end of the fourth decade (Plate 4). Plaque formation and peripheral erosion of cartilage progress to subchondral sclerosis of bone on the iliac side. The joint space contains flaky, amorphous debris. The articular capsule thickens but still permits the translatory motion noted in the second and third decades (Bowen & Cassidy 1981). Bony hypertrophy with some lipping of the sacral articular margins was noted in some specimens in the fifth decade.

The sixth and seventh decades (51–70 years)

At this stage (Figs 3.7, 3.8), the articular surfaces become totally irregular with deep erosions occasionally exposing the subchondral bone. Peripheral osteophytes enlarge and often bridge the anterior margin and inferior lip of the joint. Fibrous interconnections between the articular surfaces are commonplace; however, 'when stressed, all specimens maintained some degree of mobility, although this was restricted when compared with the younger specimens' (Bowen & Cassidy 1981). Vleeming et al (1992b) found that even in old age small movements of the sacroiliac joint are possible and ankylosis of this joint is not normal.

The eighth decade (over 70 years)

Intra-articular fibrous connections are more often the rule with some periarticular osteo-

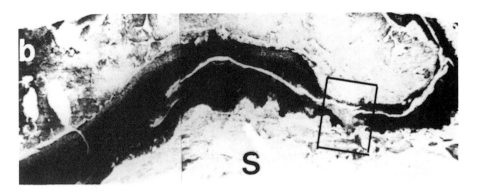

Figure 3.7 Sacroiliac joint of a male, 60 years of age. Note the variability in the depth of both the sacral (S) and the iliac cartilage at different sites. (Reproduced with permission from Walker 1986.)

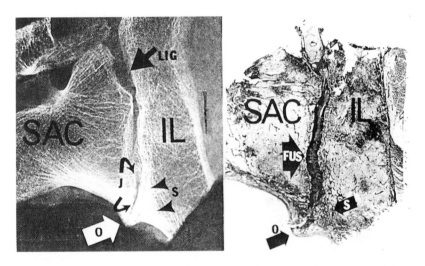

Figure 3.8 *Left*—This radiograph of a coronal section through the sacroiliac joint of a cadaver over 70 years of age illustrates narrowing of the joint space (J), sclerosis of the bone (S) and osteophyte formation (O) secondary to the degenerative process. Note the space for the interosseous ligament (LIG). *Right*—This photomicrograph reveals the thickened trabeculae in the sclerotic region (S) and an area of fibrous intra-articular fusion (FUS). (Reproduced from Resnick et al 1975, with permission of the publishers J B Lippincott.)

phytosis present (Plate 5, Fig. 3.9). Cartilaginous erosion and plaque formation is extensive and universal, filling the joint space with debris. Consequently, the joint space is markedly reduced. Intra-articular bony ankylosis is rarely reported and usually thought to be associated with ankylosing spondylitis (Fig. 3.10). Schunke (1938) reports that the average age of the specimens with bony ankylosis is considerably

less than those without fusion, confirming a probable pathological cause.

In Walker's (1986) study, 15 adult cadavers between 49 and 84 years of age were investigated for age-related changes. 'Changes observed in adult specimens were similar to those of previous reports, but from examination of the entire joint, this report emphasizes the inherent variability of the sacroiliac joint, both

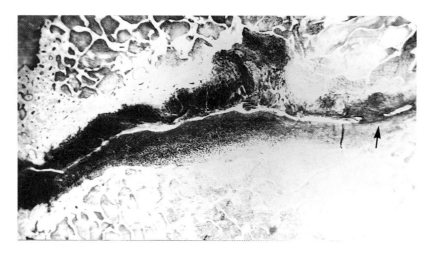

Figure 3.9 Sacroiliac joint of a female, 81 years of age. Note the erosion of the articular cartilage and the intra-articular fibrous connection (arrow). (Reproduced with permission from Walker 1986.)

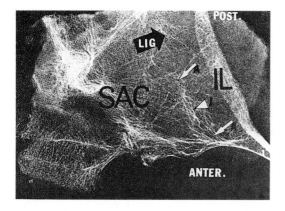

Figure 3.10 This radiograph of a transverse section through the sacroiliac joint (J, arrowhead) illustrates the intra-articular ankylosis (A, arrows) of ankylosing spondylitis. Note the ossification of the interosseous ligament (LIG). (Reproduced from Resnick et al 1975, with permission of the publishers J. B. Lippincott.)

within and between joints, at any of the ages studied.'

SUMMARY

That the sacroiliac joint degenerates with time is not unique to this articulation. The significance of this degeneration for function is unknown. Clinically, it appears that advancing age does not equate with cessation of mobility. Current evidence supports the view that the presence or absence of sacroiliac joint mobility and its significance to the patient's presenting complaints are best judged by clinical evaluation.

4

Anatomy

HISTORY

The earliest record of anatomical data pertaining to the pelvic girdle is credited to Bernhard Siegfried Albinus (1697–1770) and William Hunter (1718–1783) (Lynch 1920). These anatomists were the first to demonstrate that the sacroiliac joint was a true synovial joint, a finding confirmed by Meckel in 1816. Von Luschka, in 1854, was the first to classify the joint as diarthrodial. Further anatomical studies conducted by Albee in 1909 on 50 postmortem specimens confirmed that the joint was lined with a synovial membrane and contained by a well-formed articular capsule. His findings were confirmed by Brooke in 1924. It wasn't until 1938 (Schunke 1938) that the variations in the articular cartilage lining the iliac surface were noted. In 1957, Solonen conducted a comprehensive study of the osteology and arthrology of the pelvic girdle, from which some findings will be reported later in this chapter.

The pelvic girdle as a unit supports the abdomen and also provides a dynamic link between the vertebral column and the lower limbs. It is a closed osteoarticular ring composed of six or seven bones which include the two innominates, the sacrum, the one or two bones which together form the coccyx and the two femora, as well as six or seven joints which include the two sacroiliac, the sacrococcygeal, often an intercoccygeal, the pubic symphysis and the two hip joints.

OSTEOLOGY: THE BONES

Sacrum

Little wonder that the ancient Phallic Worshipers named the base of the spine the Sacred Bone. It is the seat of the transverse center of gravity, the keystone of the pelvis, the foundation of the spine. It is closely associated with our greatest abilities and disabilities, with our greatest romances and tragedies, our greatest pleasure and pains. (Fryette 1954)

The sacrum is a large triangular bone situated at the base of the spine wedged between the two innominates. It is formed by the fusion of five sacral vertebrae (see Fig. 3.3), and the vertebral equivalents are easily recognized. The sacrum is highly variable both between individuals and between the left and right sides of the same bone. In spite of this, certain anatomical features are consistent and only those which are essential to the description and evaluation of sacral function (Chs 5 and 7) will be described here.

The cranial aspect of the first sacral vertebra (Fig. 4.1), the sacral base, consists of the vertebral body anteriorly (the anterior projecting edge being the sacral promontory) and the vertebral arch posteriorly. Laterally, the transverse processes of the first sacral vertebra are fused with the costal elements (see Fig. 3.2) to form the alae of the sacrum. Variations have been noted (Grieve 1981) in the height of the sacral alae as

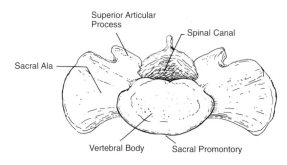

Figure 4.1 The cranial aspect of the first sacral vertebra—the sacral base.

well as the body of the S1 vertebra. The orientation of the superior articular processes of the S1 vertebra is also variable (see below).

The posterior surface of the sacrum (Fig. 4.2) is convex in both the sagittal and the transverse planes. The spinous processes of the S1 to S4 vertebrae are fused in the midline to form the median sacral crest. Lateral to the median sacral crest, the intermediate sacral crest is formed by the fused laminae of the S1 to S5 vertebrae. The laminae and inferior articular processes of the S5 (and occasionally the S4) vertebra remain unfused in the midline. They project caudally to form the sacral cornua, and together with the posterior aspect of the vertebral body of the S5 vertebra form the sacral hiatus. The lateral sacral crest represents the fused transverse processes of

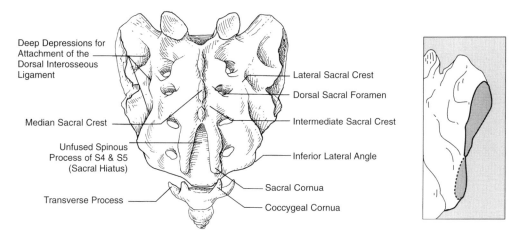

Figure 4.2 The posterior aspect of the sacrum and coccyx. *Inset*—the orientations of the three components of the articular surface resemble those of a propeller. (Redrawn from Vleeming et al 1997.)

the S1 to S5 vertebrae. Between this crest and the intermediate sacral crest lie the dorsal sacral foramina which transmit the dorsal sacral ramus of each sacral spinal nerve. There are three deep depressions in the lateral sacral crest at the levels of the S1, S2 and S3 vertebrae. These depressions contain the strong attachments of the interosseous sacroiliac ligament (Figs 4.2, 4.13).

The lateral sacral crest fuses with the costal element to form the lateral aspect of the sacrum (Fig. 4.3). Superiorly, the lateral aspect of the sacrum is wide, while inferiorly the antero-posterior dimension narrows to a thin border which curves medially to join the S5 vertebral body. This angle is called the inferior lateral angle of the sacrum (Figs 4.2, 4.4). The articular surface of the sacrum is auricular in shape (L-shaped) and is contained entirely by the costal elements of the first three sacral segments.

The short arm of the L-shaped surface (Fig. 4.3) lies in the vertical plane and is contained within the first sacral segment. The long arm lies in the anteroposterior plane within the second and third sacral segments. The contours of the articular surface are reported (Kapandji 1970, Solonen 1957, Vleeming et al 1990a, Weisl 1954, Weisl 1995) to be highly variable depending upon the age of the individual studied (see Ch. 3). Investigators have reported (Kapandji 1970) the presence of a curved furrow bordered by two longitudinal crests corresponding to a convex longitudinal crest on the articular surface of the ilium. However, Solonen (1957) in his study of 30 skeletons concluded that there were 'numerous depressions, elevations and other irregularities . . . In no case was there a distinct ridge–furrow or eminence–depression formation. On the contrary, the impression was gained that great irregularity prevails in respect to the surface formations' (Solonen 1957). His study, however, did not consider the age-related changes which may have been present in his specimens.

The anterior surface of the sacrum (Fig. 4.4) is concave in both the sagittal and the transverse planes. In the midline, four interbody ridges represent the sclerotomic fissures which are not always completely fused. Lateral to the fused vertebral bodies are four ventral sacral foramina which transmit the ventral ramus of each sacral spinal nerve as well as the segmental ventral sacral artery. The costal elements project laterally from the middle of each vertebral body between the ventral sacral foramina and fuse with those above and below as well as with the transverse processes posteriorly to form the lateral aspect of the sacrum.

The orientation of the articular surface of the sacrum in both the coronal and the transverse planes has been studied by Solonen (1957) and a summary of his findings is presented in Table 4.1. These observations represent the common

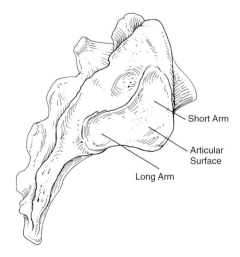

Figure 4.3 The lateral aspect of the sacrum.

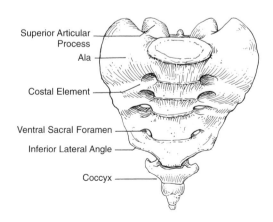

Figure 4.4 The anterior aspect of the sacrum and coccyx.

Table 4.1 Orientation of the articular surface of the sacrum in the coronal and transverse planes as described by Solonen (1957) and as shown graphically in Figure 4.5

Coronal plane	
90% of the specimens examined narrowed inferiorly at S1	Fig. 4.5A and B
85% of the specimens examined narrowed inferiorly at S2	Fig. 4.5B
80% of the specimens examined narrowed superiorly at S3	Fig. 4.5A
Transverse plane	
S1 and S2 narrow posteriorly	
S3 narrows anteriorly	

findings but variations were noted. The stereometric drawings of two pelves studied by Solonen are illustrated in Figure 4.5. Vleeming et al (Vleeming 1997) describe the orientation of the three components of the auricular surface as resembling those of a propeller (Fig. 4.2 inset).

Fryette (1954) examined 23 sacra and subsequently classified the bone into three types: A, B, and C (Figs 4.6–4.8). This classification depends on the orientation of the sacral articular surface in the coronal plane which he found to correlate with the orientation of the superior articular processes of the S1 vertebra. The Type A sacrum narrows inferiorly at S1 and S2 and superiorly at S3. The orientation of the superior articular processes in this group is in the coronal plane. The Type B sacrum narrows superiorly at S1 and the orientation of the superior articular processes in this group is in the sagittal plane. The Type C sacrum narrows inferiorly at S1 on one side (Type A) and superiorly at S1 on the other (Type B). The orientation of the superior articular processes is in the coronal plane on the Type A side and in the sagittal plane on the Type B.

In conclusion, there is a high incidence of variability in the plane of the sacroiliac joint, both in the coronal and the transverse planes as well as in the shape of the articulating surfaces. Grieve (1981) has noted that 'Each joint exhibits at least two planes slightly angulated to one another and often three—their disposition and area are not always similar when sides are compared in the same individual'. As clinicians, we are never relieved of the necessity for accurate clinical evaluation given the anatomical uncertainty of the individual being assessed.

Coccyx

The coccyx (Figs 4.2, 4.4) is represented by four fused coccygeal segments although the first is commonly separate. The bone is roughly triangular, the base bears an oval facet which articulates with the inferior aspect of the S5 vertebral body. The first coccygeal segment contains two rudimentary transverse processes as well as two coccygeal cornua which project superiorly to articulate with the sacral cornua.

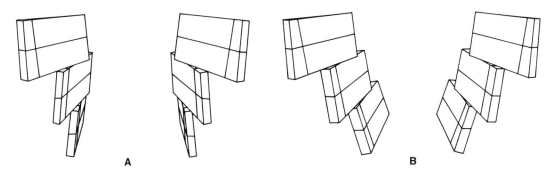

A   **B**

Figure 4.5 Stereometric drawings of two pelves studied by Solonen (1957) illustrating the variation found in the orientation of the sacral articular surface. (Redrawn with permission from Solonen 1957.)

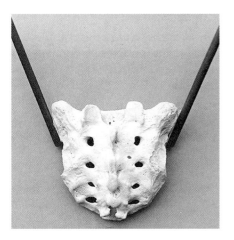
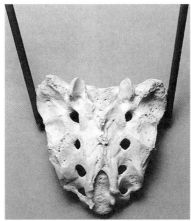
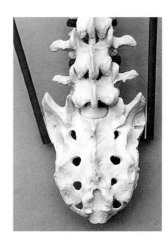

Figure 4.6

Figure 4.7

Figure 4.8

Figures 4.6 to 4.8   Sacrum types A, B and C.

Innominate

There are three parts to the innominate, the ilium, the ischium and the pubis, which in the adult are fused to form one bone, the innominate (Figs 4.9, 4.10 and see Fig. 3.4). Only the anatomical features pertinent to the description

and evaluation of function of the innominate will be described here.

Ilium

The ilium is a fan-like structure forming the superior aspect of the innominate and

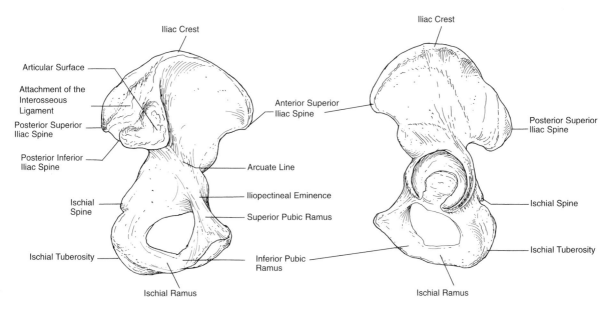

Figure 4.9

Figure 4.10

Figures 4.9 and 4.10   The medial and lateral aspects of the innominate.

contributing to the superior portion of the acetabulum. The iliac crest is convex in the sagittal plane and sinusoidal in the transverse plane such that the anterior portion is concave medially while the posterior portion is convex medially. The curve reversal occurs in the same coronal plane as the short arm of the L-shaped articular surface. The anterior superior iliac spine (ASIS) and the posterior superior iliac spine (PSIS) are at either end of the iliac crest. Inferior to the PSIS, the ilium curves irregularly to end at the posterior inferior iliac spine (PIIS). This is often the site of an accessory sacroiliac joint (Solonen 1957, Trotter 1937).

Several anatomical points are worthy of note on the medial aspect of the ilium. The articular surface lies on the posterosuperior aspect of the medial surface. Like the sacrum, the articular surface is L-shaped with the axis of the short arm in the inferosuperior plane, while the long arm has an anteroposterior axis. A variety of elevations, depressions, ridges and furrows have been reported and develop with age (see Ch. 3). Superior to the articular surface, the medial aspect of the ilium is very rough and affords attachment to the strong interosseous sacroiliac ligament which has been noted (Colachis 1963) to remain intact when the sacrum and the innominate are forced apart in cadavers. The sacroiliac joint cannot be palpated given the depth of the articulation and this point should be noted when studying the anatomy here.

Anteriorly, the arcuate line of the ilium appears at the angle between the short and the long arms of the articular surface and projects anteroinferiorly to reach the iliopectineal eminence, a point at which the ilium and the pubis unite. This line between the sacroiliac joint and the iliopectineal eminence represents a line of force transmission from the vertebral column to the lower limb and is reinforced by subperiosteal trabeculae (see Fig. 5.26) (Kapandji 1970).

Pubis

The inferomedial aspect of the innominate is formed by the pubis which articulates with the pubis of the opposite side via the pubic symphysis. It joins the ilium superiorly via the superior pubic ramus which constitutes the anterior one-fifth of the acetabulum. Inferiorly, the inferior pubic ramus projects posterolaterally to join the ischium on the medial aspect of the obturator foramen. The lateral surface of the pubis is directed towards the lower limb and affords attachment for many of the medial muscles of the thigh. The pubic tubercle is located at the lateral aspect of the pubic crest approximately 1 cm lateral to the midsymphyseal line.

Ischium

The inferolateral one-third of the innominate is formed by the ischium. The upper part of the body of the ischium forms the floor of the acetabulum as well as the posterior two-fifths of the articular surface of the hip joint. From the lower part of the body, the ischial ramus projects anteromedially to join the inferior ramus of the pubis. The ischial tuberosity is a roughened area on the posterior and inferior aspect of the ischial body and is the site of strong muscular and ligamentous attachments. Superior to the tuberosity, the ischial spine projects medially. This process is also the site of ligamentous and muscular attachments (see Figs 4.12, 4.18).

Acetabulum

The acetabulum (see Figs 4.10, 4.27) is formed from the fusion of the three bones which make up the innominate (see Fig. 3.4). It is roughly the shape of a hemisphere and projects in an anterolateral and inferior direction. The lunate surface represents the articular portion of the acetabulum while the non-articular portion constitutes the floor, or the acetabular fossa. This fossa is continuous with the acetabular notch located between the two ends of the lunate surface.

Femora

Clinically, it is important to note that the angle of inclination of the femoral neck to the shaft of the femur, as well as the angle of anteversion between the femoral neck and the coronal plane, are highly variable. This variability will be reflected in both the pattern and the range of motion available at the hip joint (Kapandji 1970).

ARTHROLOGY: THE JOINTS

Sacroiliac joint

The sacroiliac joint (Fig. 4.11) is classified as a synovial joint or diarthrosis (Bowen & Cassidy 1981). According to Bowen & Cassidy (1981) Albinus and Hunter were the first to note the presence of a synovial membrane within the joint. In 1850, Koelcher identified synovial fluid within the joint on dissection (Bowen & Cassidy 1981).

The shape, as well as the articular cartilage, have been previously described (see Ch. 3). To summarize, the sacral surface is covered with hyaline cartilage while the iliac surface is covered with a type of fibrocartilage (see Ch. 3, Plates 1–4). The depth of the articular cartilage differs both within the same articular surface and on apposing sides (see Fig. 3.7). Most investigators report (Bowen & Cassidy 1981, MacDonald & Hunt 1951, Solonen 1957) a ratio of 1:3 between the iliac and sacral surfaces.

The joint capsule is composed of two layers, an external fibrous layer which contains abundant fibroblasts, blood vessels and collagen fibers and an inner synovial layer. The chronological changes in the articular capsule have been described (Ch. 3). Anteriorly, the capsule is clearly distinguished from the overlying ventral sacroiliac ligament, while posteriorly the fibers of the capsule and the deep interosseous ligament are intimately blended. Inferiorly, the capsule blends with the periosteum of the contiguous sacrum and innominates.

Like other synovial joints, the sacroiliac joint capsule is supported by overlying ligaments and fascia, some of which are the strongest in the body. They include the:

1. ventral sacroiliac ligament
2. interosseous sacroiliac ligament
3. long dorsal sacroiliac ligament
4. sacrotuberous ligament
5. sacrospinous ligament
6. iliolumbar ligament
7. thoracodorsal fascia.

Ventral sacroiliac ligament

The ventral sacroiliac ligament (Fig. 4.12) is the weakest of the group and is little more than a thickening of the anterior and inferior parts of the joint capsule (Bowen & Cassidy 1981, Warwick & Williams 1989). Clinically, when the sacroiliac joint is hypermobile (see Ch. 9), this ligament is invariably attenuated and often a source of pain. The ligament can be palpated anteriorly at Baer's point (see Ch. 7). When it is responsible for the patient's complaints, the pain can be reproduced or magnified by palpation as well as by stressing this structure (see Ch. 7, transverse anterior distraction/posterior compression pain provocation test and Fig. 7.34).

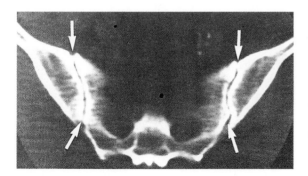
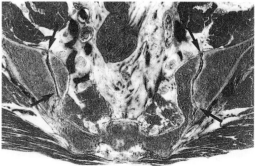

Figure 4.11 A computed tomography scan (left) with a photograph of the corresponding anatomical section (right) through the synovial portion of a cadaveric sacroiliac joint (arrows). (Reproduced from Lawson et al 1982 with permission of the publishers Raven Press.)

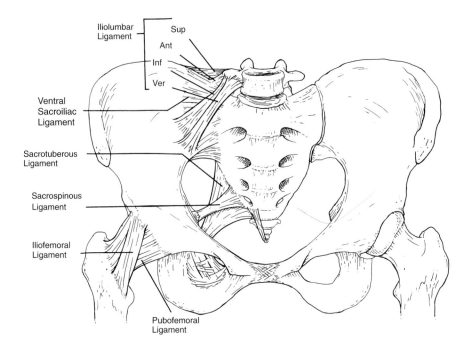

Figure 4.12 The ligaments of the pelvic girdle viewed from the anterior aspect.

Interosseous sacroiliac ligament

The interosseous sacroiliac ligament is the strongest of the group and completely fills the space between the lateral sacral crest and the iliac tuberosity (Fig. 4.13 and see Fig. 3.8). The fibers are multidirectional and can be divided into a deep and a superficial group. The deep layer attaches medially to three fossae on the lateral aspect of the dorsal sacral surface (see Fig. 4.2) and laterally to the adjacent iliac tuberosity. The superficial layer of this ligament is a fibrous sheet which attaches to the lateral sacral crest at S1 and S2 and to the medial aspect of the iliac crest. This structure is the primary barrier to direct palpation of the sacroiliac joint in its superior part and its density makes intra-articular injections extremely difficult.

Long dorsal sacroiliac ligament

The dorsal sacroiliac ligament (Fig. 4.14) attaches medially to the lateral sacral crest at S3 and S4

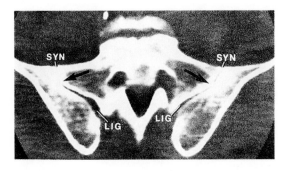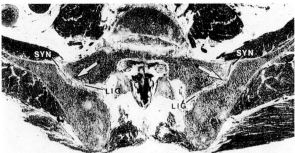

Figure 4.13 A computed tomography scan (left) with a photograph of the corresponding anatomical section (right) through the sacroiliac joint. Note the depth of the synovial portion (SYN) of the joint and the interosseous ligament (LIG). (Reproduced from Lawson et al 1982 with permission of the publishers Raven Press.)

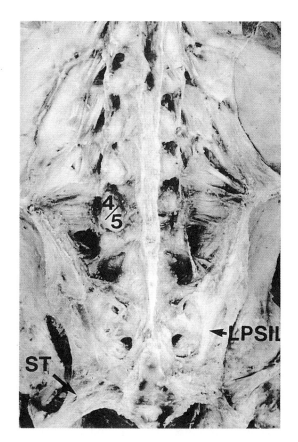

Figure 4.14 A dorsal view of the female pelvic girdle. LPSIL is the long dorsal SI ligament, 4/5 is the zygapophyseal joint between L4 and L5, ST is the sacrotuberous ligament. (Reproduced from Willard 1997 with permission of the publishers Churchill Livingstone.)

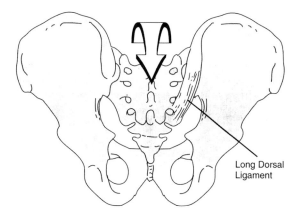

Figure 4.15 Counternutation of the sacrum tightens the long dorsal ligament. This increase in tension can be palpated just inferior to the posterior superior iliac spine (PSIS). (Redrawn from Vleeming et al 1996.)

Tension can be increased in this ligament during motion of the sacrum and contraction of the muscles which blend with it. During counternutation of the sacrum, the ligament tightens (Fig. 4.15) (Vleeming et al 1996). During nutation of the sacrum, the ligament relaxes. Contraction of the erector spinae muscle as well as loading of the sacrotuberous ligament will also increase tension in this ligament, whereas contraction of the latissimus dorsi and the gluteus maximus muscles has been found to reduce the tension (Vleeming et al 1997).

The skin overlying the ligament is a frequent area of pain in patients with lumbosacral and pelvic girdle dysfunction (Fortin et al 1994a, 1994b, 1997). Tenderness on palpation of the long dorsal sacroiliac ligament does not necessarily incriminate this tissue, given the nature of pain referral both from the lumbar spine and the sacroiliac joint.

Sacrotuberous ligament

This ligament is composed of three large fibrous bands, the lateral, medial and superior (Fig. 4.16) (Willard 1997). The lateral band connects the ischial tuberosity and the posterior inferior iliac spine and spans the piriformis muscle from which it receives some fibers. The medial band attaches to the transverse tubercles of S3, S4 and S5 and the lateral margin of the lower sacrum

and laterally to the posterior superior iliac spine and the inner lip of the iliac crest. It lies posterior to the interosseous ligament and is separated from it by the emerging dorsal branches of the sacral spinal nerves and blood vessels. It can be palpated directly caudal to the PSIS as a thick band and at this point it is covered by the fascia of the gluteus maximus muscle. Medially, fibers of this ligament attach to the deep lamina of the posterior layer of the thoracolumbar fascia and the aponeurosis of the erector spinae muscle (Vleeming et al 1996). At a deeper level, connections have been noted between the long dorsal ligament and the multifidus muscle (Willard 1997). Laterally, fibers blend with the superior band of the sacrotuberous ligament.

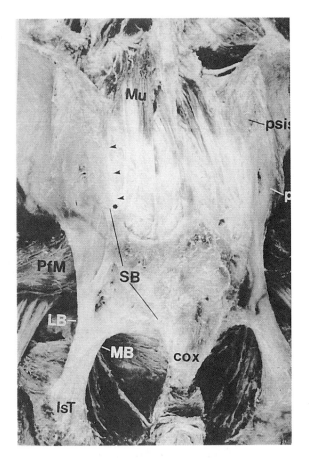

Figure 4.16 A dorsal view of the male pelvic girdle, ligaments intact and all but the deepest laminae of multifidus (Mu) removed. The arrowheads mark the long dorsal ligament beneath the lateral band (LB) of the sacrotuberous ligament which arches over the piriformis muscle (PfM). The medial band (MB) of the sacrotuberous ligament traverses the ischial tuberosity (IsT) and the coccyx. The superior band of the sacrotuberous ligament (SB) runs superficial to the long dorsal ligament to connect the coccyx with the PSIS. Tendons of the multifidus (Mu) pass between the superior band and the long dorsal ligament to insert into the body of the sacrotuberous ligament. The asterisk marks the transverse tuberosity of the lateral sacral crest. (Reproduced from Willard 1997 with permission of the publishers Churchill Livingstone.)

and coccyx. These fibers run anteroinfero-laterally to reach the ischial tuberosity. The fibers of this band spiral, such that those arising from the lateral aspect of the ischial tuberosity insert into the caudal part of the sacrum while those from the medial aspect of the ischial tuberosity attach cranially (Vleeming et al 1996). The superior band runs superficial to the interosseus

ligament and connects the coccyx with the PSIS. The gluteus maximus also attaches to the sacrotuberous ligament and its contraction can increase the tension in the sacrotuberous ligament (Vleeming et al 1989a,b).

Phylogenetically, the sacrotuberous ligament represents the tendinous insertion of the biceps femoris muscle in lower vertebrates (Warwick & Williams 1989). In some humans, this ligament still receives some fibers from the biceps femoris muscle (Fig. 4.17) (Vleeming et al 1989a, 1995b). The fibers of the biceps femoris muscle can bridge the ischial tuberosity completely to attach directly into the sacrotuberous ligament.

The tendons of the deep laminae of the multifidus muscle can also blend into the superior surface of the sacrotuberous ligament (Fig. 4.16) (Willard 1997). The ligament is pierced by the perforating cutaneous nerve (S2, S3) which subsequently winds around the inferior border of the gluteus maximus muscle to supply the skin covering the medial and inferior part of the buttock, perhaps a source of paraesthesia when entrapped.

Sacrospinous ligament

The sacrospinous ligament (Figs 4.12, 4.18) attaches medially to the lower, lateral aspect of the sacrum and the coccyx. Laterally, the apex of this triangular ligament attaches to the ischial spine of the innominate. Proximally, fibers blend with the capsule of the sacroiliac joint (Willard 1997). It is closely connected to the coccygeus muscle of which it may represent a degenerated part (Warwick & Williams 1989). Clinically, this ligament may be responsible for the secondary coccydynia experienced by patients with pelvic girdle dysfunction.

Iliolumbar ligament

Bogduk (1997) continues to describe five bands of the iliolumbar ligament: anterior, superior, inferior, vertical (Fig. 4.12) and posterior (Fig. 4.19). The anterior band attaches to the anteroinferior aspect of the entire length of the transverse process of the L5 vertebra. It blends with the superior band anterior to the quadratus

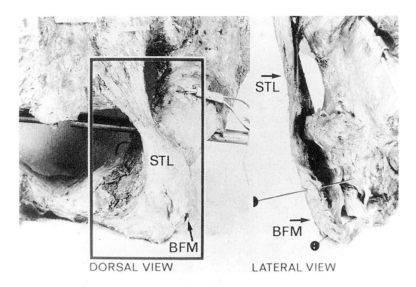

STL

STL

BFM

BFM

DORSAL VIEW   LATERAL VIEW

Figure 4.17   The biceps femoris muscle (BFM) has been found to alter tension in the sacrotuberous ligament (STL) through its indirect (attaching to the ischial tuberosity first), and in some, direct (bypassing the ischial tuberosity) connection to the ligament. (Reproduced with permission from Vleeming et al 1995b.)

lumborum muscle to attach to the anterior margin of the iliac crest. The superior band arises from the tip of the transverse process of the L5 vertebra. Laterally, the band divides to envelop the quadratus lumborum muscle before inserting onto the iliac crest. The posterior band also arises from the tip of the transverse process of the L5 vertebra. Laterally, it inserts onto the iliac tuberosity posteroinferiorly to the superior band. The inferior band arises both from the body and

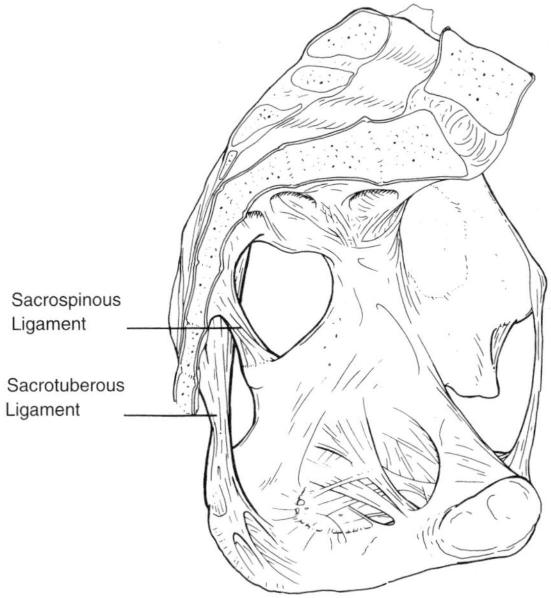

Sacrospinous
Ligament

Sacrotuberous
Ligament

Posterior Band
(Iliolumbar Ligament)

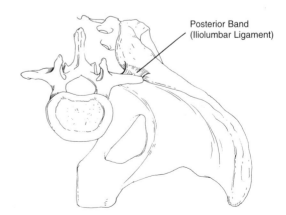

Figure 4.18   A sagittal section of the pelvic girdle illustrating the anchoring effect of the sacrotuberous ligament on the sacral base.

Figure 4.19   A transverse section of the lumbosacral junction illustrating the attachment of the posterior band of the iliolumbar ligament.

the inferior border of the transverse process of the L5 vertebra. Inferiorly, the fibers cross the ventral sacroiliac ligament obliquely to attach to the iliac fossa. The vertical band arises from the anteroinferior border of the transverse process of the L5 vertebra. These fibers descend vertically to attach to the posterior aspect of the arcuate line.

Willard (1997) reports that the individual bands of the iliolumbar ligament are highly variable in number and form, but consistently arise from the transverse processes of the L4 and L5 vertebrae blending inferiorly with the sacroiliac ligaments and laterally with the iliac crest. Previous descriptions of the evolution of this ligament from the quadratus lumborum muscle in the second decade of life (Luk et al 1986) have been refuted with the discovery of this ligament in the fetus (Uhtoff 1993, Hanson & Sonesson 1994).

Both Bogduk (1997) and Willard (1997) speculate that these ligaments are responsible for maintaining the stability of the lumbosacral junction both in the coronal and the sagittal planes.

Thoracodorsal fascia

The thoracodorsal fascia is a critical structure when considering transference of load from the trunk to the lower extremity (Vleeming et al 1995a). Several muscles, important in providing stability to the pelvic girdle, attach to this fascia and can affect tension within it. They include the transversus abdominis, internal oblique, gluteus maximus, latissimus dorsi, erector spinae, multifidus and biceps femoris.

Its anatomy is complex. There are three layers to the fascia, the anterior, middle and posterior. The anterior layer is thin (Bogduk 1997) and covers the anterior aspect of the quadratus lumborum muscles. It attaches medially to the transverse processes and blends with the intertransverse ligaments. The middle layer is posterior to the quadratus lumborum. It arises medially from the tips of the transverse processes and provides origin to the aponeurosis of the transversus abdominis.

There are two laminae which comprise the posterior layer of the thoracodorsal fascia. The superficial lamina is predominantly derived from the aponeurosis of the latissimus dorsi muscle (Fig. 4.20) and contains oblique fibers which run caudomedially. In the midline, strong connections exist to attach the fascia to the supraspinal ligaments and the spinous processes of the lumbar vertebrae cranial to L4. According to Willard (1997), the posterior border of the ligamentum flavum becomes the supraspinous ligament, which in turn is anchored to the thoracodorsal fascia (Figs 4.21, 4.22). Through these attachments, tension of the thoracodorsal

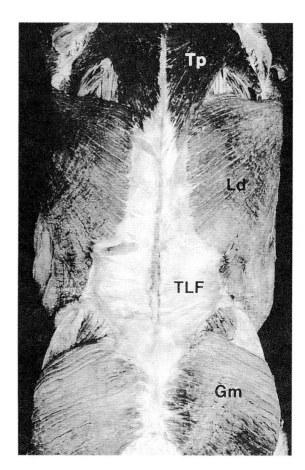

Figure 4.20 A posterior view of the thoracodorsal fascia (also known as the thoracolumbar fascia—TLF) illustrates the attachments of latissimus dorsi (Ld) and gluteus maximus (Gm) into the superficial lamina of the posterior layer. Note the small attachment of the lower fibers of the trapezius muscle (Tp). (Reproduced from Willard 1997 with permission of the publishers Churchill Livingstone.)

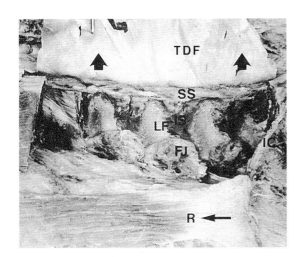

Figure 4.21 Dorsolateral view of the lumbar spine. The left iliac crest (IC) is exposed. The arrow points rostral (R) to facilitate orientation of this dissection. The thoracodorsal fascia (TDF) blends with the supraspinous ligament (SS) and interspinous ligament (IS), ligamentum flavum (LF) and the facet joint (FJ) capsule. (Reproduced from Willard 1997 with permission of the publishers Churchill Livingstone.)

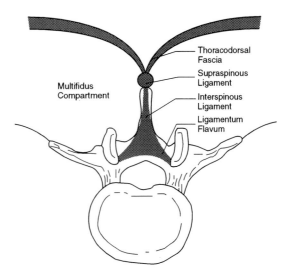

Figure 4.22 Horizontal view of the lumbar region illustrating the ligamentum flavum/interspinous ligament/supraspinous ligament/thoracodorsal fascia connections. This mechanism plays a significant role in stabilization training of the lumbo-pelvic-hip region. (Redrawn from Williard 1997 with permission of the publishers Churchill Livingstone.)

fascia is transmitted to the ligamentum flavum and, according to Willard (1997), assists in the alignment of the lumbar vertebrae. The superficial laminae also receives some fibers from the external oblique and the lower trapezius muscles (Vleeming et al 1995a).

Caudal to L4, midline connections are very loose and actually cross the midline to reach the opposite iliac crest and sacrum. Over the sacrum, the superficial lamina blends with the fascia of the gluteus maximus. These fibers run in a caudolateral direction from a medial attachment to the median sacral crest and occasionally as far cranial as the L4 spinous process (Fig. 4.23).

The deep lamina of the posterior layer of the thoracodorsal fascia is also complex with several muscular connections (Fig. 4.24). The fibers run in a caudolateral direction attaching medially to the interspinous ligaments and caudally to the PSIS, iliac crest and posterior sacroiliac ligaments. Above the pelvis, the deep lamina attaches to the lateral raphe and blends with the middle layer of the thoracolumbar fascia. The internal oblique and the transversus abdominis muscles attach to this lateral raphe. Over the pelvis, some fibers blend with the deep fascia of the erector spinae muscle and the sacrotuberous ligament.

Tension of the thoracodorsal fascia can be increased through motion of the arms, trunk and lower extremity. Contraction or lengthening of the many muscles which attach into the fascia can influence its tension. In this manner, stability of the pelvic girdle and low back is enhanced and load is effectively transferred from the trunk to the lower extremity.

Sacrococcygeal joint

The sacrococcygeal joint is classified as a symphysis although synovial joints have been found at this articulation. Maigne (1997) examined nine specimens and found one fibrocartilaginous disc, four synovial joints and four mixed (part synovial and part fibrocartilaginous). All of the specimens were older and it is not known if the sacrococcygeal joint can change from one form to another during a lifetime. The supporting ligaments include the ventral sacrococcygeal ligament, dorsal sacro-

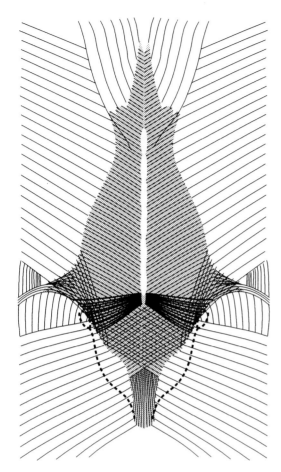

Figure 4.23 The superficial lamina of the thoracodorsal fascia. (Redrawn from Vleeming et al 1997 with permission of the publishers Churchill Livingstone.)

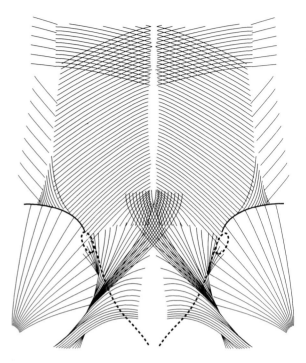

Figure 4.24 The deep lamina of the thoracodorsal fascia. (Redrawn from Vleeming et al 1997 with permission of the publishers Churchill Livingstone.)

Intercoccygeal joint

The intercoccygeal joint is classified as a symphysis in the young since the first two segments are separated via a fibrocartilaginous disc. With time, the joint usually ossifies; however, it occasionally remains synovial.

Pubic symphysis

This joint contains a fibrocartilaginous disc (Fig. 4.25a), has no synovial tissue nor fluid, and therefore is classified as a symphysis. The osseous surfaces are covered by a thin layer of hyaline cartilage; however, they are separated by the fibrocartilaginous disc. The posterosuperior aspect of the disc often contains a cavity which is not seen before the age of 10 years (Warwick & Williams 1989). This is a non-synovial cavity and may represent a chronological degenerative change. The supporting ligaments of this articulation (Figs 4.25a, b, c) include the superior

coccygeal ligament and the lateral sacrococcygeal ligament.

The ventral sacrococcygeal ligament represents the continuation of the anterior longitudinal ligament of the vertebral column. The dorsal sacrococcygeal ligament has two layers. The deep layer attaches to the posterior aspect of the body of the S5 vertebra and the coccyx (analogous to the posterior longitudinal ligament), whereas the superficial layer bridges the margins of the sacral hiatus and the posterior aspect of the coccyx, thus completing the sacral canal. Laterally, the intercornual ligaments, or the lateral sacrococcygeal ligaments, connect the sacral and coccygeal cornua.

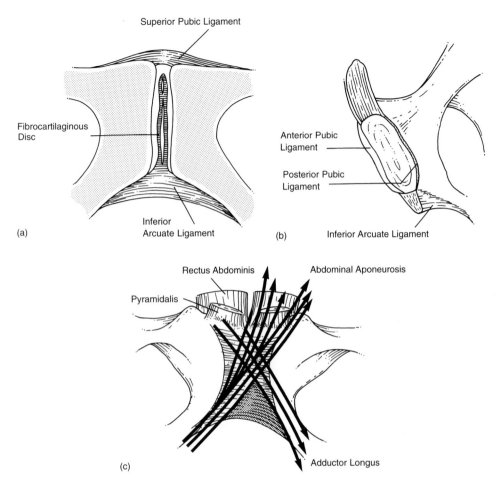

Figure 4.25 The pubic symphysis. (a) A coronal section. (b) A sagittal section through the fibrocartilaginous disc. (c) The anterior aspect. (Redrawn from Kapandji 1974.)

pubic ligament, inferior arcuate ligament, posterior pubic ligament and the anterior pubic ligament.

The superior pubic ligament is a thick fibrous band which runs transversely between the pubic tubercles of the pubic bones. Inferiorly, the arcuate ligament blends with the fibrocartilaginous disc to attach to the inferior pubic rami bilaterally. The posterior pubic ligament (Fig. 4.25b) is membranous and blends with the adjacent periosteum while the anterior ligament of the pubic symphysis is very thick and contains both transverse and oblique fibers (Kapandji 1974). It receives fibers from the aponeurotic expansion of the abdominal musculature as well

as the adductor longus muscle which decussates across the joint (Fig. 4.25c).

Hip joint

The hip joint (Fig. 4.26) is classified as an unmodified ovoid synovial joint (MacConaill & Basmajian 1977). The head of the femur forms roughly two-thirds of a sphere, and except for a small fovea it is covered by hyaline cartilage which decreases in depth toward the periphery of the surface. The acetabulum has been described (see Osteology section). The lunate surface of the acetabulum (Fig. 4.27) is lined with hyaline cartilage while the non-articular portion,

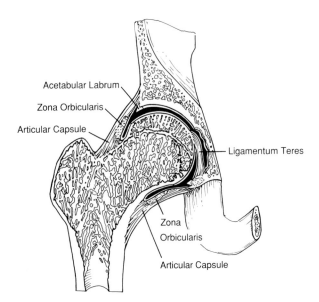

Figure 4.26   A coronal section through the hip joint.

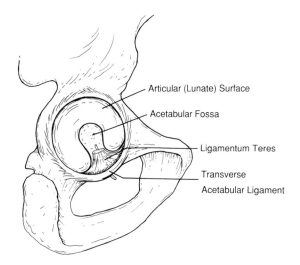

Figure 4.27   The acetabulum.

the acetabular fossa, is filled with loose areolar tissue and covered with synovium. The acetabulum is deepened by a fibrocartilaginous labrum which on cross-section is triangular in shape. The base of the labrum attaches to the rim of the acetabulum except inferiorly where it is deficient at the acetabular notch, which is bridged by the transverse acetabular ligament. The apex of the labrum is lined with articular

cartilage and lies inside the hip joint as a free border; the capsule of the joint attaches to the labrum at its peripheral base, thus creating a circular recess.

The articular capsule encloses the joint and most of the femoral neck. Medially, it attaches to the base of the acetabular labrum and extends 5 to 6 cm beyond this point onto the innominate. Inferiorly, the medial attachment is to the transverse acetabular ligament. Laterally, the capsule inserts onto the femur anteriorly along the entire extent of the trochanteric line, posteriorly to the femoral neck above the trochanteric crest, superiorly to the base of the femoral neck and inferiorly to the femoral neck above the lesser trochanter. The superficial bands of the capsular fibers are predominantly longitudinal while the deep bands are circular forming the zona orbicularis (Fig. 4.26) which has few, if any, osseous connections. The zona orbicularis divides the synovial cavity into a medial and a lateral recess. The ligaments which are intimately blended with, and support, the capsule include the iliofemoral ligament, pubofemoral ligament, and the ischiofemoral ligament. There are two intra-articular ligaments, the ligamentum teres and the transverse acetabular ligament.

Iliofemoral ligament

The iliofemoral ligament (Figs 4.12, 4.28, 4.29) is extremely strong and reinforces the anterior aspect of the hip joint. It is triangular in shape and attaches to the anterior inferior iliac spine at its apex. Inferolaterally, it diverges into two bands, the lateral iliotrochanteric band which inserts onto the superior aspect of the trochanteric line and the medial inferior band which inserts onto the inferior aspect of the trochanteric line. Together, these two bands form an inverted Y, the center of which is filled with weaker ligamentous tissue.

Pubofemoral ligament

The pubofemoral ligament (Figs 4.12, 4.28) attaches medially to the iliopectineal eminence

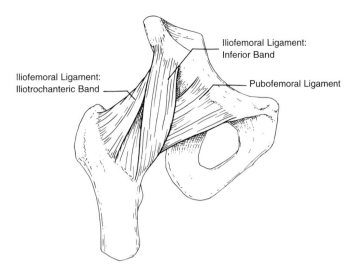

Figure 4.28   The ligaments of the anterior aspect of the hip joint.

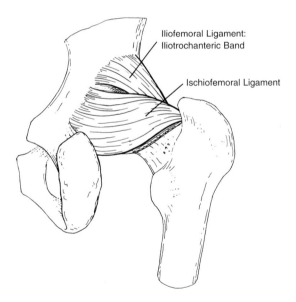

Figure 4.29   The ligaments of the posterior aspect of the hip joint.

the psoas major muscle crosses the joint at this point contributing to its dynamic support. A bursa is located here between the tendon of the psoas muscle and the capsule and occasionally will communicate directly with the synovial cavity of the hip joint.

Ischiofemoral ligament

The ischiofemoral ligament (Fig. 4.29) arises medially from the posterior aspect of the acetabulum and its labrum. Laterally, the fibers spiral superoanteriorly over the back of the femoral neck to insert anterior to the trochanteric fossa deep to the iliofemoral ligament. Some fibers from this ligament also run transversely to blend with those forming the zona orbicularis.

Ligamentum teres

The ligamentum teres (Figs 4.26, 4.27) attaches laterally to the anterosuperior part of the fovea of the femoral head and medially via three bands to either end of the lunate surface of the acetabulum inferiorly and to the upper border of the transverse acetabular ligament.

and the superior pubic ramus as well as to the obturator crest and membrane. Laterally, it attaches to the anterior surface of the trochanteric line. The capsule of the hip joint is unsupported by any ligament between the pubofemoral ligament and the inferior band of the iliofemoral ligament; however, the tendon of

Transverse acetabular ligament

This ligament is a continuation of the acetabular labrum inferiorly and converts the acetabular notch into a foramen through which the intra-articular vessels pass to supply the head of the femur (Fig. 4.27).

In addition to the ligamentous support, the hip joint is dynamically stabilized by numerous muscles including the iliacus, rectus femoris, pectineus, gluteus minimus, piriformis, obturator externus, obturator internus, superior and inferior gemellus muscles as well as the fascia lata of the thigh, all of which partially insert into the articular capsule.

MYOLOGY: THE MUSCLES

There are 35 muscles which attach directly to the sacrum and/or innominate and function with the ligaments and fascia to produce synchronous motion and stability of the trunk and the extremities. They include the following:

1. latissimus dorsi
2. external oblique
3. internal oblique
4. transverse abdominis
5. rectus abdominis
6. pyramidalis
7. gluteus medius
8. gluteus minimus
9. gluteus maximus
10. piriformis
11. superior gemellus
12. inferior gemellus
13. obturator internus
14. obturator externus
15. semimembranosus
16. semitendinosus
17. biceps femoris
18. quadratus femoris
19. adductor brevis
20. adductor longus
21. adductor magnus
22. pectineus
23. gracilus
24. rectus femoris
25. sartorius
26. tensor fascia lata
27. erector spinae
28. quadratus lumborum
29. iliacus
30. psoas minor
31. levator ani
32. sphincter urethrae
33. superficial transverse perineal and ischiocavernosus
34. coccygeus
35. multifidus.

Although 'Classic myology, with its emphasis on origins and insertions, often fails to convey the dynamism of an active contracting structure exerting a force between its two fixed ends' (Farfan 1978), some anatomical review is required to facilitate the subsequent discussion of biomechanics and clinical syndromes. Later, some of these muscles will be discussed with respect to their role in providing stability to the pelvic girdle. The reader should refer to a good anatomy text for detail on the muscles listed but not described below.

Multifidus

The deepest fibers of the multifidus muscle in the lumbar spine (the laminar fibers) arise from the posteroinferior aspect of the lamina and articular capsule of the zygapophyseal joint and insert onto the mammillary process (Bogduk 1997) of the level below. The remainder of the muscle arises medially from the spinous process, blending laterally with the laminar fibers. Inferiorly, the fascicles insert *three* levels below, such that those arising from the L1 vertebra insert onto the mammillary processes of the L4, L5 and S1 vertebrae as well as the medial aspect of the iliac crest. Inferiorly, the fibers from the spinous process of the L2 vertebra insert onto the mammillary processes of the L5 and S1 vertebrae and the PSIS of the innominate. The fibers from the spinous process of the L3 vertebra insert onto the S1 articular process, the superolateral aspect (costal element) of the S1 and S2 segments and the iliac crest. The fibers from the spinous process of the L4 vertebra insert onto the lateral sacral crest and the area of bone between this crest and the dorsal sacral foramina, while those from the L5 vertebra insert onto the intermediate sacral crest inferiorly to S3. Within the pelvis, the multifidus muscle also attaches to the deep laminae of the posterior thoracodorsal fascia at a raphe which separates it from the gluteus maximus muscle (Willard 1997). Here, fibers from the multifidus pass beneath the posterior sacroiliac ligaments to blend with the sacrotuberous ligament (Fig. 4.16). The interconnections of the multifidus muscle facilitate its contribution to stability of the low back and pelvis.

The fascicles are innervated by the medial branch of the dorsal ramus such that all of the fascicles which arise from the same spinous process are innervated by the same nerve regardless of the inferior extent of their insertion (Bogduk 1983, 1997).

Erector spinae

Lumbar longissimus

This muscle (Fig. 4.30) arises from five muscle laminae, the deepest of which is from the L5 vertebra overlapped by those from L4, then L3, then L2 and finally L1 (Bogduk 1997). Medially, these laminae arise from the segmental transverse and accessory processes. Laterally, the fibers from the L1 to L4 vertebrae insert via a common tendon into the medial aspect of the lumbar intermuscular aponeurosis which attaches inferiorly to the PSIS of the innominate. The fibers from the L5 vertebra pass more posteriorly than inferiorly in comparison to the fibers from the L1 vertebra which pass more inferiorly than posteriorly to insert onto the medial aspect of the PSIS. Consequently, the lower fibers can act unilaterally as segmental rotators and bilaterally as posterior translators. Clinically, the lower fibers may be responsible for producing the lumbar kyphosis, or rotoscoliosis, seen in patients with an acute L5–S1 joint dysfunction. A myofascial etiology could explain the rapid restoration of the lumbar lordosis following treatment with neuromuscular inhibition techniques (Grieve 1986).

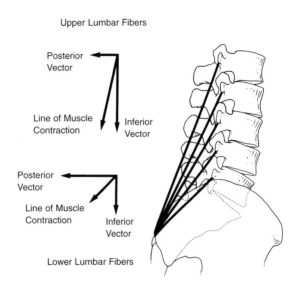

Figure 4.30 The lumbar longissimus muscle. Note the relative posterior orientation of the fibers from the L5 vertebra as opposed to the inferior orientation of the fibers from the L1 vertebra. The force vectors which occur as a result of contraction of the muscle are depicted on the left. The lower lumbar fibers have a greater posterior 'pull' than the upper lumbar fibers which have a greater inferior 'pull'. (Redrawn from Bogduk 1997.)

Lumbar iliocostalis

This muscle (Fig. 4.31) arises as four overlapping laminae from the tips of the transverse processes of the L1 to L4 vertebrae. Inferiorly, the muscle inserts onto the PSIS and the superior aspect of the iliac crest 3 to 5 cm lateral to the PSIS. The inferior laminae from the L4 vertebra have a more posterior orientation than the superior fibers from the L1 vertebra. Bogduk (1980, 1997) notes that this muscle is a more effective rotator than the lumbar longissimus muscle since its attachment is further lateral on the transverse process, and hence has a longer lever arm.

Thoracic longissimus and thoracic iliocostalis

According to Bogduk (1997) these two muscles are not confined to the thorax but span several segments to gain attachment both to the PSIS of the innominate and to the aponeurosis of the erector spinae muscle, which covers the lumbar longissimus muscle before attaching to the

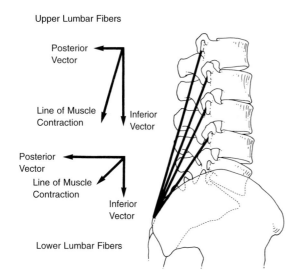

Figure 4.31 The lumbar iliocostalis muscle. Note the relative posterior orientation of the lower fibers and the omission of attachment to the L5 vertebra. The force vectors which occur as a result of contraction of the muscle are depicted on the left. The lower lumbar fibers have a greater posterior 'pull' than the upper lumbar fibers which have a greater inferior 'pull'. (Redrawn from Bogduk 1997.)

posteroinferior aspect of the sacrum. Consequently, these muscles are also capable of influencing the motion of bones which do not directly articulate.

Quadratus lumborum

A pertinent point to note here is the attachment of this muscle to the superior and anterior bands of the iliolumbar ligament (Bogduk 1997, Luk et al 1986). This muscle may contribute to the dynamic stability of the lumbosacral junction by increasing the tension of the iliolumbar ligament.

Gluteus maximus

This muscle is the largest in the body and attaches extensively to the pelvic girdle. It arises from the posterior gluteal line of the innominate, the dorsum of the lower lateral sacrum and coccyx, the aponeurosis of erector spinae muscle, the sacrotuberous ligament, the superficial

laminae of the posterior thoracodorsal fascia and the fascia covering the gluteus medius muscle. In the pelvis, the gluteus maximus blends with the ipsilateral multifidus through the raphe of the thoracodorsal fascia (Willard 1997) and the contralateral latissimus dorsi through the superficial laminae of the thoracodorsal fascia (Fig. 4.20) (Vleeming et al 1995a).

Less than one-half of this muscle attaches directly to the gluteal tuberosity of the femur. The remainder inserts into the iliotibial tract of the fascia lata (Farfan 1978).

Piriformis

The piriformis muscle arises from the anterior aspect of the S2, S3 and S4 segments of the sacrum as well as the capsule of the sacroiliac joint, the anterior aspect of the PIIS of the ilium, and often the upper part of the sacrotuberous ligament. Its exit from the pelvis is through the greater sciatic foramen (see Fig. 6.1) and it attaches to the greater trochanter of the femur.

This muscle is important in stabilization of the sacroiliac joint; however too much tension can be responsible for restricting sacroiliac joint motion and/or producing local pain (McQueen 1977, Mitchell 1965, Travell & Rinzler 1952). Entrapment neuropathies of the sciatic nerve as it passes through and/or beneath the piriformis muscle can occur. Trigger points located in this muscle as well as the gluteus medius, longissimus and multifidus muscles have been reported to refer pain to the sacroiliac joint (Travell & Rinzler 1952).

With regard to a piriformis syndrome (Kirkaldy-Willis & Hill 1979, McQueen 1977, Maxwell 1978, Mennell 1952, Mixter & Barr 1934), Grieve (1981) notes:

Because muscle tenderness of itself has not engendered elsewhere in the body a host of muscle syndromes like trapezius syndrome, deltoid syndrome, sacrospinalis syndrome, gluteal syndrome, gastrocnemius syndrome and so on, it may appear somewhat indiscriminative to attach such importance to the name of a tender muscle as to propose a clinical entity on the basis of what is almost certainly a 2° [secondary] consequence.

Rectus abdominis

A key point to note concerning this muscle is the inferior attachment to the pubic symphysis. The aponeurotic expansions of this muscle, along with those of the transversus abdominis, internal oblique, pyramidalis and adductor longus muscles, interdigitate anterior to the symphysis to form a dense network of fibers and thus contribute to the stability of this articulation (see Fig. 4.25c) (Kapandji 1974, Warwick & Williams 1989).

Pyramidalis

This triangular muscle is located anterior to the inferior aspect of the rectus abdominis muscle and is enclosed within its sheath. The base attaches to the os pubis as well as to the symphysis while the apex blends with the linea alba midway between the umbilicus and the pubis. This muscle is innervated by the subcostal nerve which is the ventral ramus of the T12 spinal nerve. Clinically, superoinferior asymmetry of the pubic symphysis can be effectively treated by restoring the function of the T12–L1 spinal segment. Perhaps the pyramidalis muscle, via altered neurophysiology from the T12–L1 spinal segment, is responsible for maintaining the clinically observed positional asymmetry of the pubic symphysis.

External oblique

The external oblique is the largest and most superficial of the abdominal muscles. It arises from eight digitations from the external and inferior surfaces of the lower eight ribs. The upper attachments are close to the costal cartilages, the lowest is to the apex of the 12th rib and those in-between form an oblique line between these two points. The fibers diverge inferomedially, the posterior ones almost vertically to attach to the outer lip of the anterior half of the iliac crest. The upper and middle fibers are progressively less oblique and insert into a complex anterior aponeurosis. Rizk (1980) investigated this structure in 41 specimens and

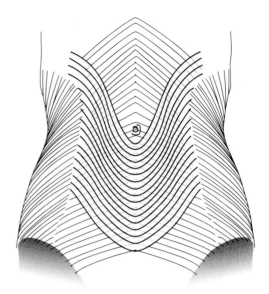

Figure 4.32 The deep and superficial fibers of the anterior abdominal fascia cross the midline to blend with those of the opposite side in a similar manner to the posterior layer of the thoracodorsal fascia.

discovered that the aponeurosis of the external oblique was bilaminar. The orientation of the two layers is similar to the posterior layer of the thoracodorsal fascia in that the fibers from both layers cross the midline to blend with the fascia of the opposite side. The deep and superficial layers produce a cross-hatched appearance as their orientations are 90° to each another (Fig. 4.32).

Internal oblique

The internal oblique lies between the external oblique and the transversus abdominis and arises from the lateral two-thirds of the inguinal ligament, anterior two-thirds of the intermediate line of the iliac crest and to the lateral raphe of the thoracodorsal fascia. The posterior fibers ascend laterally to reach the tips of the 11th and 12th ribs and the 10th rib near the costochondral junction. The anterior fibers arising from the inguinal ligament arch inferomedially to blend with the aponeurosis of transversus abdominis and attach to the pubic crest. The intermediate fibers pass superomedially to insert into a bilaminar aponeurosis (Rizk 1980), blending with the aponeurosis of the external oblique forming a decussating network of fascia across the midline of the body.

Transversus abdominis

The transversus abdominis is the deepest abdominal muscle and arises from the lateral one-third of the inguinal ligament, the anterior two-thirds of the inner lip of the iliac crest, the lateral raphe of the thoracodorsal fascia and the internal aspect of the lower six costal cartilages interdigitating with the costal fibers of the diaphragm. From this broad attachment, the muscle runs transversely around the trunk where its upper and middle fibres blend with the fascial envelope of the rectus abdominis reaching the linea alba in the midline (Fig. 4.33). Inferiorly, the muscle blends with the insertion of the internal oblique muscle to reach the pubic crest.

Levator ani

This muscle forms the pelvic floor. It can be divided into four parts: puborectalis, pubococcygeus, iliococcygeus and ischiococcygeus. Anteriorly, the puborectalis and pubococcygeus attach to the body of the pubis and the anterior part of the obturator fascia. The puborectalis passes posteriorly lateral to the urethra, vagina

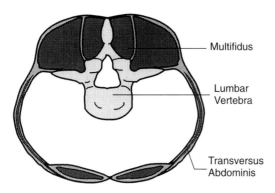

Figure 4.33 The transversus abdominis runs transversely around the trunk to attach to the fascial envelope of the rectus abdominis anteriorly and the lateral raphe of the thoracodorsal fascia posteriorly. (Reproduced from Richardson et al 1996.)

(females) and rectum to unite with its counterpart to form a muscular sling at the anorectal flexure; there is no posterior osseous attachment. The pubococcygeus passes posteriorly, inferior to the puborectalis, and attaches to a midline raphe posterior to the rectum. Through this raphe, fibers unite and continue posteriorly from the anorectal flexure to attach to the anterior aspect of the last two coccygeal segments. The iliococcygeus and ischiococcygeus (coccygeus) arise from the medial aspect of the ischial spine, the posterior part of the obturator fascia and the medial aspect of the sacrospinous ligament. Fibers from these muscles complete the pelvic floor and attach to the anterior aspect of the apex of the sacrum at S5.

Though rarely reported spontaneously, a common subjective complaint in patients with pelvic girdle dysfunction is pain during sexual intercourse and/or defecation. This muscle can be responsible, if the pelvic girdle asymmetry is sufficient to alter the muscle's resting length.

Iliacus

The iliacus muscle arises from the iliac fossa, the ventral sacroiliac ligament and the inferior fibers of the iliolumbar ligament (Bogduk 1997) as well as the lateral part (costal element) of the sacrum. Distally, its fibers converge to merge with the lateral aspect of the tendon of the psoas muscle while some go on to insert directly onto the lesser trochanter of the femur. As it crosses the hip joint, some fibers attach to the upper part of the capsule.

Psoas minor

This muscle is absent in 40% of the population and when present arises from the sides of the bodies of the T12 and L1 vertebrae as well as the intervertebral disc (Warwick & Williams 1989). Distally, it inserts onto the iliopectineal eminence of the innominate. It is supplied by the ventral ramus of the L1 spinal nerve.

Psoas major

Although this muscle does not directly attach to either the innominate or the sacrum, its influence

Labels in figure: Multifidus, Lumbar Vertebra, Transversus Abdominis on the biomechanics of the region is significant. The muscle attaches to the anteroinferior border of the transverse processes of the L1 to L5 vertebrae as well as to the intervertebral discs and adjacent vertebral bodies. Medially, it blends with the tendinous arch which spans the waist of each vertebral body beneath which pass the segmental nerves and blood vessels.

Inferiorly, the muscle fibers converge into a tendon which receives the iliacus muscle medially before crossing the anterior aspect of the hip joint between the iliofemoral and pubofemoral ligaments. Inferiorly, the tendon inserts onto the lesser trochanter of the femur. The tendon is separated from the capsule of the hip joint by the iliopsoas bursa. The muscle is innervated via the ventral rami of the L1 and L2 spinal nerves, and hence the neurophysiological connection to the thoracolumbar junction.

The fascia of the leg

The fascia of the lower extremity envelops the muscles and via its extensive attachments to the pelvic girdle can influence its function and subsequently become symptomatic in dysfunction. The fascia encircles the pelvic girdle by attaching to the sacrum, coccyx, iliac crest, inguinal ligament, superior pubic ramus, inferior pubic ramus, ischial ramus, ischial tuberosity and sacrotuberous ligament. Superiorly, it blends with the thoracolumbar and abdominal fascia of the trunk. From the iliac crest, the fascia descends over the gluteus medius muscle before splitting to envelop the gluteus maximus muscle. The two bands meet at the lower border of this muscle and facilitate its insertion into the iliotibial tract which represents a lateral thickening of the fascia.

The iliotibial tract attaches inferiorly to the condyles of the femur and the tibia, and to the head of the fibula blending with the crural fascia and aponeurotic extensions of the quadriceps muscle. The fascia is continuous in the thigh with two intermuscular septa which attach to the linea aspera.

The tensor fascia lata muscle inserts into the iliotibial tract anterior to the attachment of the gluteus maximus muscle. This muscle is also enveloped by two layers of the fascia. The superficial layer reaches the iliac crest lateral to the muscle while the deep layer blends medially with the capsule of the hip joint.

NEUROLOGY: THE NERVES

Understanding the neurology of the lumbo-pelvic-hip region is essential since rehabilitation involves the restoration of optimal neurological function. Muscle control in posture and locomotion depends directly on both the central and peripheral nervous systems. Janda (1986) notes that 'It is almost impossible clinically to differentiate the primary changes in muscle from their secondary reaction due to an altered or impaired central nervous regulation, as the quality of muscle function depends directly on the central nervous system activity'.

Wyke (1981, 1985) has shown that articular neurology has both direct and reflex influences on muscle tone locally and globally. In addition, afferent input from articular structures contributes to perception of posture and motion. Altered afferent input from the articular mechanoreceptors can have profound influences on both static and dynamic pelvic girdle function.

Macroscopic articular neurology

Rudinger (1857) is reported (Solonen 1957) to be the first to describe the macroscopic innervation of the sacroiliac joint. The subject has still not been investigated extensively, especially histologically.

The most extensive study of the macroscopic innervation of the sacroiliac joint was done in 1957 by Solonen. He examined 18 joints in nine cadavers and found that posteriorly all of the joints were innervated from branches of the posterior rami of the S1 and S2 spinal nerves. Bradlay (1985) reported that the dorsal sacroiliac ligaments, and presumably the joint, receive supply from the lateral divisions of the dorsal rami of the L5, S1, S2 and S3 spinal nerves. The lateral branches of the L5, S1 and S2 dorsal rami form a plexus between the dorsal sacroiliac and interosseous ligaments from which the joint is innervated. This was later confirmed by Grob et al (1995).

Anteriorly, Solonen (1957) found that the articular innervation was not always consistent nor necessarily symmetrical. Of the 18 specimens examined, all of the joints were innervated by branches from the ventral rami of the L5 spinal nerve, 17 from L4, 11 from S1, 4 from S2, 1 from L3 and 15 received innervation from the superior gluteal nerve. Grob et al (1995) were unable to confirm any innervation from the ventral rami. The wide distribution of innervation is reflected clinically in the variety of pain patterns reported by patients with sacroiliac joint dysfunction (Fortin 1994a).

The hip joint is innervated by branches from the obturator nerve (L2, L3, L4), the nerve to the quadratus femoris (L2, L3, L4) and the superior gluteal nerve (L5, S1) (Grieve 1986). As well, the joint receives branches from the nerves which supply the muscles crossing the joint. The hip joint is principally derived from the L3 segment of mesoderm with contributions from L2 to S1; hence the potential for a variety of patterns of pain referral.

The outer one-third of the lumbar intervertebral disc is innervated posteriorly by the sinuvertebral nerve (Bogduk 1983, 1997) and laterally by the ventral rami and gray rami communicantes of the spinal nerve. Nociceptors (see below) have been located here, thus the anatomical potential for primary disc pain. The zygapophyseal joints of the L5 and S1 vertebrae are innervated via the medial branch of the dorsal ramus of the L4, L5 and S1 spinal nerves.

Microscopic articular neurology

Accurate information from mechanoreceptors in the joint is required by the central nervous system so that the activity of the motor units essential for position, motion and stability of the joint is coordinated. This mechanism protects the joint from excessive motion and coordinates the timing of motor recruitment such that habitual movements are produced in an efficient and biomechanically safe manner.

There is more than one classification of joint receptors (Rowinski 1985, Wyke 1981). Essentially, there are receptors in all layers of the capsule, in all ligaments and fascia and within all parts of the muscles. Some have a low threshold for discharge and are slow in adapting. They report on static position of the joint, muscle length and tone and intra-articular pressure. Others have a low threshold for discharge and adapt very quickly. These receptors report dynamic changes in the environment including changes in joint position (direction, quantity and velocity). The receptors which have a high threshold for discharge adapt very slowly and are protective. The effect of these receptors is to reflexively inhibit further muscle contraction and prevent further stretch of the joint capsule.

Nociceptors are located throughout the articular and myofascial system. They respond to extremes of mechanical deformation and/or chemical irritation (potassium ions, lactic acid, polypeptide kinins, 5-hydroxytryptamine, acetylcholine, noradrenalin, prostaglandins, histamine) and are high threshold, non-adapting receptors. These receptors contribute to the perception of pain (nociception); however, the afferent input can be significantly altered both peripherally and centrally.

According to Wyke (1981) the central effects of articular mechanoreceptor activity are threefold: reflex, perceptual and pain suppression.

Reflex effects. Depolarization of the afferent fibers from the low threshold articular mechanoreceptors reaches the fusimotor neurons polysynaptically, thus contributing to the gamma feedback loop from the muscle spindle both at rest and during joint motion. 'By this means the articular mechanoreceptors exert reciprocally coordinated reflexogenic influences on muscle tone and on the excitability of stretch reflexes in all the striated muscles' (Wyke 1981). When this capsular reflex is activated, the discharging receptors facilitate the muscles antagonistic to the occurring movement. When the high threshold articular mechanoreceptors are discharged, the reflex effect is projected polysynaptically to the alphamotoneurons and results in local muscular inhibition. Nociceptors effect the discharge from the alpha-motoneurone pool and can distort the normal, coordinated, mechanoreceptor reflex system (Gandevia 1992).

Perceptual effects. Afferent input from the articular mechanoreceptors travels polysynaptically via the posterior and dorsal spinal columns to reach the paracentral and parietal regions of the cerebral cortex, thus contributing significantly, though not solely, to both postural and kinesthetic awareness.

The observation that capsulectomy of the hip joint performed in the course of hip replacement surgery does not result in total loss of postural sensation at the hip, leaves no doubt that while joint capsule mechanoreceptors contribute to awareness of static joint position, they are not the sole source of perceptual experience, and other recent studies suggest that their contribution in this regard is supplementary to and coordinated with that provided by the inputs from cutaneous and myotatic [muscle spindle] mechanoreceptors!' (Wyke 1981)

Pain. According to Grieve (1981):

No matter where it is felt in the body, and no matter from what cause, pain—which is the commonest of all clinical symptoms encountered in medical practice—represents a disturbance of neurological function.

Unlike taste, touch or smell, pain is not a primary neurological sensation but rather a complex neurological phenomenon influenced by patterns of activity in specific afferent systems as well as by past and present experiences.

Impulses subserving pain are not transmitted centrally by small-diameter fibers only. The entire spectrum of afferent fibers may be stimulated by peripheral noxious stimuli, depending upon the intensity of the stimulus. The experience of pain depends upon mechanisms of convergence, summation and modulation both peripherally in the spinal cord and centrally in the brain stem and cortex.

The theory of peripheral modulation, or spinal gating, was originally proposed by Melzak & Wall (1965). Briefly, the gate-control mechanism depends on large fiber activity (mechanoreceptor) which presynaptically inhibits the transmission of impulses from the small fiber nociceptors at the substantia gelatinosa. Thus 'by rhythmic movement of the body, or a body part, and by cutaneous contact and soft tissue compression, i.e. stroking, holding and by rhythmic manual or mechanical mobilization techniques, the large diameter (6–12 microns and 13–17 microns) mechanoreceptors are stimulated' (Grieve 1981) and subsequently modulate the transmission of nociceptor activity.

Centrally, the perception of pain can be influenced by psychological factors including past experience, anxiety and culture, and drugs such as caffeine, alcohol and barbiturates, all of which increase the experience of pain.

Muscular neurology

The peripheral nerves and their spinal root derivatives which innervate the muscles of the pelvic girdle are found in Table 4.2.

ANGIOLOGY: THE BLOOD SUPPLY

The hip joint is supplied by the obturator, the medial and lateral femoral circumflex and the superior and inferior gluteal arteries and veins (Crock 1980, Grieve 1983, Singleton & LeVeau 1975). The acetabular fossa, its contents as well as the head of the femur, receive supply from the acetabular branch of the obturator and medial femoral circumflex vessels via the ligamentum teres (see Fig. 4.27). The vascular anatomy is inconsistent and rarely sufficient to sustain the viability of the head of the femur following interruption of other sources of supply.

Experimental findings (Astrom 1975) point to a connection between aching pain, elevation of intraosseous pressure and impaired [venous] drainage of spongiosa. Rhythmic mobilizations of this articulation are extremely effective in relieving persistent aches associated with osteoarthritis. Together with the effects of mechanoreceptor discharge during these techniques perhaps improved circulation plays a role in pain suppression. (Grieve 1983)

The nutrient arteries and veins for the sacrum arise from the lateral and median sacral system. The lateral sacral vessels arise from the posterior trunk of the internal iliac and descend over the anterolateral aspect of the sacrum. The two

Table 4.2   The peripheral nerves and their spinal root derivatives which innervate the muscles of the pelvic girdle

Muscle	Peripheral nerve	Roots
Abdominals	Ventral rami	T12, L1
Pyramidalis	Subcostal nerve	T12
Gluteus medius	Superior gluteal	L5, S1
Gluteus minimus	Superior gluteal	L5, S1
Gluteus maximus	Inferior gluteal	L5, S1, S2
Piriformis	Ventral rami	L5, S1, S2
Superior gemellus	Nerve to obturator internus	L5, S1
Inferior gemellus	Nerve to quadratus femoris	L5, S1
Obturator externus	Obturator	L3, L4
Obturator internus	Nerve to obturator internus	L5, S1
Quadratus femoris	Nerve to quadratus femoris	L5, S1
Semimembranosus	Tibial	L5, S1, S2
Semitendinosus	Tibial	L5, S1, S2
Biceps femoris	Tibial, common peroneal	L5, S1, S2
Adductor brevis	Obturator	L2, L3, L4
Adductor longus	Obturator	L2, L3, L4
Adductor magnus	Obturator, tibial	L2, L3, L4
Pectineus	Femoral, accessory obturator	L2, L3
Gracilus	Obturator	L2, L3
Rectus femoris	Femoral	L2, L3, L4
Sartorius	Femoral	L2, L3
Tensor fascia lata	Superior gluteal	L4, L5
Erector spinae	Lateral and intermediate branches of the segmental dorsal rami	
Quadratus lumborum	Ventral rami	T12–L3(4)
Iliacus	Femoral	L2, L3, L4
Psoas minor	Ventral rami	L1
Levator ani	Inferior rectal, pudendal	S4
Sphincter urethra	Perineal branch pudendal	S2, S3, S4
Coccygeus	Ventral rami	S4, S5
Multifidus	Medial branch of segmental dorsal ramus	
Psoas major	Ventral rami	L1, L2, L3

longitudinal arteries give off anterior central branches which course medially to anastomose with the median sacral artery. The anterior central branches send feeder vessels into the centrum of the sacrum. At the level of the ventral sacral foramina, spinal branches supply the cauda equina as well as the contents of the sacral canal. The foraminal branch, after passing through the dorsal sacral foramina, supplies the posterior aspect of the medial and intermediate sacral crests as well as the posterior musculature. Venous drainage is via vessels which accompany the arteries and subsequently drain into the common iliac system.

The nutrient supply for the innominate is derived from the iliac branches of the obturator and iliolumbar vessels as well as the superior gluteal vessels (Warwick & Williams 1989).

5

Biomechanics of the lumbo-pelvic-hip complex

The primary function of the lower quadrant is to move and to simultaneously provide a stable base from which the upper extremity can function. Together, the trunk and the lower extremities have the potential for multidimensional movement with a minimum of energy expenditure (Abitbol 1995, 1997, McNeill Alexander 1995, 1997). Neuromusculoskeletal harmony is essential for optimal lumbo-pelvic-hip function. Meisenbach in 1911 stated that:

> When the trunk is moved to one side quickly there are direct opposing forces of the lumbar and spinal muscles against the pelvic and leg muscles. Normally these work in harmony and are resisted by the strong pelvic ligaments and fascia to a certain extent. If the harmony of these muscles is disturbed from some cause or another, or if the ligamentous support is weakened, other points of fixation must necessarily yield.

It is traditional to study both anatomy and biomechanics in a regional manner. For example, the lumbar spine is often considered separately from the pelvic girdle which in turn is investigated separately from the hip. This approach yields information as to how the parts function but not as to how the parts work together. While it is necessary to consider the function of the individual parts, rehabilitation is unsuccessful without consideration of how these parts achieve the harmonious action noted by Meisenbach 87 years ago. After studying individually the biomechanics of the lumbar spine, pelvic girdle and hip, the collective biomechanics will be presented. Hopefully, a more integrated perspective of both the anatomy and biomechanics of the lumbo-pelvic-hip region can be achieved. First, a description of the terminology used is required.

TERMINOLOGY

The terms kinematics (the study of movement) and kinetics (the study of forces) come from the science of kinesiology, the study of biomechanics (Table 5.1). The prefixes osteo-, arthro-and myo- are Greek derivatives meaning bone, joint and muscle respectively.

Osteokinematics refers to the study of motion of bones regardless of the motion of the joints.

All bones move at joints. But the kinematics of a bone does not require any inquiry into the kinematics of the joint at which the bone moves. The bone is considered simply as an object moving in space, an object that can be studied without opening the joint. (MacConaill & Basmajian 1977)

These motions are named according to the axis about which they occur.

Flexion/extension occurs when one or more bones rotate about a coronal axis. This terminology is consistent throughout the spinal column and peripheral joints. Currently, the accepted terms for flexion and extension of the sacrum are nutation and counternutation respectively. Forward rotation of the innominate about a coronal axis is termed anterior rotation, backward rotation is termed posterior rotation. Abduction/adduction occurs when one or more

appendicular (peripheral) bones rotate about a sagittal axis. Sideflexion occurs when an axial bone (skull, vertebral column) rotates about a sagittal axis. Medial/lateral rotation occurs when one or more appendicular (peripheral) bones rotate about a vertical or longitudinal axis. Axial rotation occurs when an axial bone (skull, vertebral column) rotates about a vertical or longitudinal axis. The bones can also translate along the same axes resulting in posteroanterior, anteroposterior, mediolateral, lateromedial and vertical (distraction–compression) translation.

When the trunk bends forward/backward in a sagittal plane about a coronal axis, this is called forward/backward bending. A sideways motion in the coronal plane about a sagittal axis is called lateral bending. A twist of the body about a vertical plane is called axial rotation.

Arthrokinematics refers to the study of motion of joints regardless of the motion of the bones. 'Intra-articular kinematics or arthrokinematics has to do with the movement of one articular surface upon another ... Articular surfaces can spin and/or slide upon each other' (MacConaill & Basmajian 1977). These motions are referred to as pure spins and pure and impure swings. A pure spin occurs when the only motion of a point on the articular surface is a rotation around the mechanical axis of the bone. A pure swing occurs when the only motion of a point on the articular surface is a slide along the shortest possible line (the chord) between two points. An impure swing occurs when a point on the articular surface slides along any other curved line (an arc) between two points such that an element of spin also occurs.

Myokinematics refers to the study of motion of bones produced by the contraction of the muscle. 'Myokinematics has to do with the way in which the structure and arrangement of a set of muscle fibers determines the amount of angular motion associated with its full contraction, and so the range of movement it can help to occur' (MacConaill & Basmajian 1977).

Osteokinetics, arthrokinetics and myokinetics refer to the study of forces met by the bones, joints and muscles during static and dynamic function.

Table 5.1 Definition of biomechanical terms (Warwick & Williams 1989)

Term	Definition
Kinematics	The study of motion of particles and rigid bodies without consideration of the forces involved
Kinetics	The study of the effects of forces on the motion of materials
Osteo-	Bone
Arthro-	Joint
Myo-	Muscle

KINEMATICS OF THE LUMBO-PELVIC-HIP REGION

Kinematics of the lumbar spine

Newton's second law states that the motion of an object is directly proportional to the applied force and occurs in the direction of the straight line in which the force acts. Translation occurs when a single net force causes all points of the object to move in the same direction over the same distance (Bogduk 1997). Rotation occurs when two unaligned and opposite forces cause the object to move around a stationary center or axis (Bogduk 1997). In mechanical terms, the lumbar vertebrae have the potential for 12 degrees of freedom (Levin 1997) (Fig. 5.1), as motion can occur in a positive and negative direction along and about three perpendicular axes.

However, this model does not account for the anatomical factors which modify and restrict the actual motion which can occur. Clinically, the lumbosacral junction appears to exhibit four degrees of freedom of motion (Bogduk 1997, Pearcy & Tibrewal 1984, Vicenzino & Twomey 1993).

1. flexion coupled with posteroanterior translation
2. extension coupled with anteroposterior translation
3. right sideflexion/rotation coupled with mediolateral translation
4. left sideflexion/rotation coupled with mediolateral translation.

Flexion/extension is an integral part of forward/backward bending of the trunk while rotation/sideflexion occurs during any other motion of the trunk.

Flexion/posteroanterior translation and extension/anteroposterior translation

Flexion/posteroanterior translation (Fig. 5.2) of the lumbar spine occurs during forward bending of the trunk. The coronal axis is

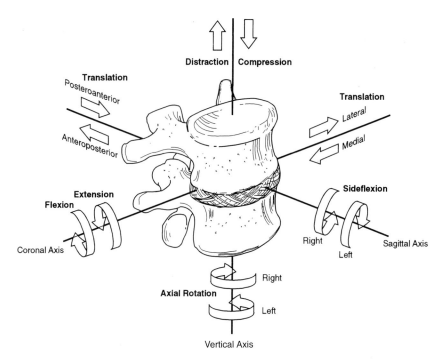

Figure 5.1 In mechanical terms, there is the potential for 12 degrees of motion of the lumbar vertebrae (Bogduk 1997, Levin 1997).

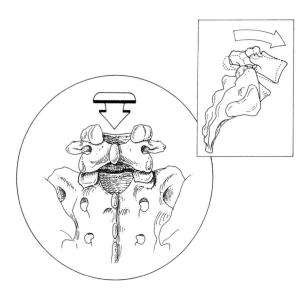

Figure 5.2 Flexion/posteroanterior translation at L5–S1.

dynamic rather than static and moves forward with flexion such that flexion couples with a small degree (1–3 mm) of anterior translation (Figs 5.2, 5.3) (Bogduk 1997, Gracovetsky & Farfan 1986, Gracovetsky et al 1981, White & Panjabi 1978). Extension/anteroposterior translation of the lumbar spine occurs during backward bending of the trunk.

The arthrokinematics which occur at the zygapophyseal joints during flexion and extension are impure swings. During flexion, the

inferior articular processes of the superior vertebra glide superiorly and anteriorly along the superior articular processes of the inferior vertebra/sacrum (Bogduk 1997). During extension, the inferior articular processes of the superior vertebra glide inferiorly and posteriorly along the superior articular processes of the inferior vertebra/sacrum. The total amplitude of this glide is about 5–7 mm.

Rotation/sideflexion

Motion coupling of the vertebral column during rotation or lateral bending of the trunk was first recorded by Lovett in 1903. He noted that a flexible rod bent in one plane could not bend in another without twisting. The direction of this motion coupling has been a controversial issue.

In 1984, Pearcy & Tibrewal reported on a three-dimensional radiographic study of lumbar motion during rotation and lateral bending of 10 men under 30 years of age. Their findings of coupled motion (Fig. 5.4) were consistent with those of Gracovetsky & Farfan (1986) except at the lumbosacral junction where if lateral bending occurred, it was always in the same direction as the axial rotation. L4–L5 was noted to be transitional following the movement pattern of either L3–L4 or L5–S1. Rotation/sideflexion was very restricted at the lumbosacral

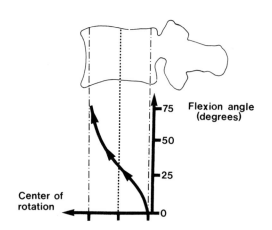

Figure 5.3 The coronal axis for flexion/extension moves anteriorly with increasing degrees of flexion.

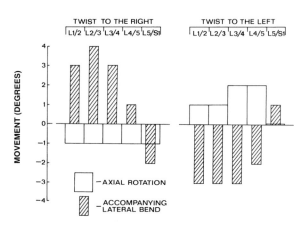

Figure 5.4 Findings of coupled motion of rotation and lateral bending in the lumbar spine. At the lumbosacral junction, lateral bending occurs in the same direction as the induced rotation. (Redrawn from Pearcy & Tibrewal 1984.)

junction when compared to the other levels. This study did not investigate the coupling of motion when lateral bending was introduced from a position of flexion or extension.

According to Bogduk (1997), *pure* axial rotation of a lumbar motion segment is possible up to 3°. At this point, all of the fibers of the annulus fibrosus that are aligned in the direction of the rotation are under stress, the contralateral zygapophyseal joint is compressed in its sagittal component and the ipsilateral zygapophyseal joint capsule is under tension. The initial axis for this motion is vertical through the posterior part of the vertebral body. After 3° of rotation, the axis shifts to the impacted zygapophyseal joint and the upper vertebra pivots about this new axis. The vertebral body swings posterolaterally imposing a lateral translation force on the intervertebral disc. The impacted inferior articular process swings backwards and medially further stretching the capsule and ligaments. Further rotation can result in failure of any of the stressed or compressed components. According to Bogduk (1997), 35% of the resistance to torsion is provided by the intervertebral disc and 65% by the posterior elements of the neural arch.

Bogduk (1997) supports Pearcy & Tibrewal's (1984) model of motion coupling and concurs that for the upper three segments axial rotation is accompanied by contralateral sideflexion. This motion is unidirectional about an oblique axis and also involves slight flexion or extension of the segment (Fig. 5.5). He agrees that at L5–S1 the pattern tends to be ipsilateral (Fig. 5.6) and that L4–5 is variable. In addition, he notes that individual variation exists and resists any rules for segmental motion patterning.

While recognising these patterns, it is important to note that they represent average patterns. Not all individuals exhibit the same degree of coupling at any segment or necessarily in the same direction as the average; nor do all normal individuals necessarily exhibit the average direction of coupling at every segment.

Vicenzino & Twomey (1993) investigated the conjunct rotation which occurred during lateral bending of the lumbar spine and noted that in 64% of their specimens no conjunct rotation

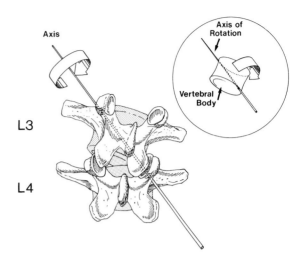

Figure 5.5 Left rotation of the L3–L4 joint complex couples with contralateral sideflexion and slight flexion or extension.

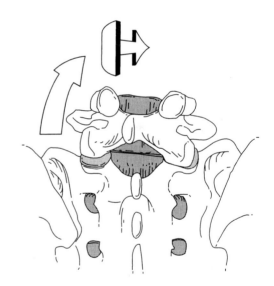

Figure 5.6 During right rotation, the L5 vertebra rotates/sideflexes to the right.

occurred at L5–S1. In the remainder, the direction of rotation was always the same as sideflexion. This coupling of motion was consistent when the segment was sideflexed from a flexed, neutral or extended position. Above L5–S1 an interesting pattern emerged. In extension, L1–2 and L3–4 rotated opposite to the direction of sideflexion. In flexion, L1–2 and

L3–4 rotated in the same direction as the sideflexion. Conversely, in extension, L2–3 and L4–5 rotated in the same direction as the sideflexion and in flexion L2–3 and L4–5 rotated in the opposite direction! The conclusion from this study was that the coupling of motion in the lumbar spine was indeed complex.

The biomechanics of the lumbosacral junction have been shown (Farfan 1973, Gilmore 1986, Grieve 1986, Kirkaldy-Willis 1983, Kirkaldy-Willis et al 1978, Stokes 1986, Twomey & Taylor 1986, White & Panjabi 1978) to change with both age and degeneration. The instantaneous center of rotation for flexion/extension and/or rotation/sideflexion can be significantly displaced with degeneration, resulting in excessive posteroanterior and/or lateral translation during physiological motion of the trunk (Stokes 1986, White & Panjabi 1978.) Consequently, 'on the intersegmental level … normal loads may in fact be acting about a displaced IAR [instantaneous axis of rotation], thus locally producing abnormal motion' (Gilmore 1986).

In summary, even if the biomechanics of the lumbosacral junction were confirmed and conclusive, the potential for altered biomechanics to exist is high, rendering 'perceptive clinical observation of a patient [as] the most direct way to assess spine motion clinically, despite its lack of objectivity' (Stokes 1986).

Kinematics of the pelvic girdle

Mobility of the sacroiliac joint has been recognized since the 17th century. Since the middle of the 19th century, both postmortem and in vivo studies have been done in an attempt to clarify the movements of the sacroiliac joints and the pubic symphysis and the axes about which these movements occur (Albee 1909, Colachis et al 1963, Egund et al 1978, Goldthwait & Osgood 1905, Kissling & Jacob 1997, Lavignolle et al 1983, Meyer 1878, Miller et al 1987, Sashin 1930, Sturesson et al 1989, 1997, Walheim & Selvik 1984, Weisl 1954, 1955, Wilder et al 1980, Vleeming et al 1990a,b).

The investigative methods include: manual manipulation of the sacroiliac joint both at surgery and in a cadaver (Chamberlain 1930, Fothergill 1896, Jarcho 1929, Lavignolle et al 1983); X-ray analysis in various postures of the trunk and lower extremity (Albee 1909, Brooke 1924); roentgen stereophotogrammetric and stereoradiographic imaging after the insertion of tantalum balls into the innominate and sacrum (Egund et al 1978, Sturesson et al 1989, 1997, Walheim & Selvik 1984); inclinometer measurements in various postures of the trunk and lower extremity, after the insertion of Kirschner wires into the innominate and sacrum (Colachis et al 1963, Kissling & Jacob 1997, Pitkin & Pheasant 1936), and computerized analysis using a Metrecom Skeletal Analysis System (Smidt 1995). Clinical theories (DonTigny 1985, 1990, 1997, Hesch et al 1992, 1997, Lee 1989, 1992) have also contributed significantly towards the research in this region. The results of these studies have led to proposals concerning both function and dysfunction of the pelvic girdle.

The following section will detail the current status concerning both the known and the proposed biomechanics of the pelvic girdle. The model incorporates the findings of research and clinical impressions.

Motion of the pelvis itself can occur in all three body planes: flexion/extension in the sagittal plane during forward and backward bending, sideflexion in the coronal plane during lateral bending and axial rotation in the transverse plane during twisting of the trunk. A combination of all of these motions occurs during the normal gait cycle (Greenman 1990, 1997). During these habitual movements, motion also occurs within the pelvis. While sacroiliac joint mobility is normally very limited, movement has been shown to occur (Miller et al 1987, Sturesson et al 1989, 1997, Walheim & Selvik 1984) throughout life (Vleeming et al 1992b, 1997).

Until recently, the quantity of motion present has been debated. In 1983, Lavignolle et al reported 10–12° of posterior rotation of the innominate coupled with 6 mm of anterior translation, and 2° of anterior rotation coupled with 8 mm of anterior translation, in an in vivo study of two women and three men under 25 years of age. This study was conducted in the non-weight bearing position and Vleeming et al (1990a) note that this is probably a significant factor in the quantity of motion reported. Sturesson et al (1989) used roentgen stereophoto-grammetric analysis (RSA) to investigate sacroiliac joint mobility in 21 women from 19 to 45 years of age and four men from 18 to 45 years of age. They found only 2.5° of innominate rotation and 0.5–1.6 mm of translation. This in vivo study was conducted in the weight-bearing position. Sturesson et al felt that the other authors (Colachis et al 1963, Lavignolle et al 1983, Weisl 1954, 1955) had overestimated the mobility of the sacroiliac joint.

Jacob & Kissling's (1995) findings of sacroiliac joint mobility using the RSA technique supported those of Sturesson et al (1989). The average values for rotation and translation were low, being 1.8° of rotation and 0.7 mm of translation for the men and 1.9° of rotation and 0.9 mm translation for the women. No statistical differences were noted for either age or gender. They postulated that more than 6° of rotation and 2 mm of translation should be considered pathologic (Jacob & Kissling 1995).

Nutation/counternutation of the sacrum

Motion at the sacroiliac joint occurs during movements of the trunk and the lower extremity. Sacral nutation is the forward motion of the sacral promontory into the pelvis about a coronal axis within the interosseous ligament (Fig. 5.7). This motion occurs bilaterally when moving from supine lying to standing and increases slightly during the initial stages of forward bending of the trunk. Unilateral sacral nutation occurs during flexion of the lower extremity. Sacral counternutation is the backward motion of the sacral promontory about a coronal axis within the interosseous ligament (Fig. 4.15) and occurs bilaterally when lying supine and in some towards the end of forward bending of the trunk. Unilateral counternutation of the sacrum occurs during extension of the lower extremity. This is an osteokinematic description of how the bones of the pelvic girdle move in relation to one another.

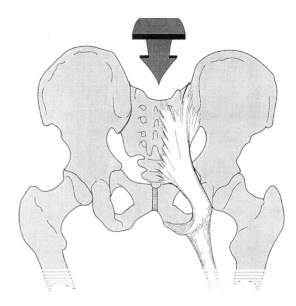

Figure 5.7   Sacral nutation is the forward motion of the sacral promontory into the pelvis. This motion is resisted by the interosseous and sacrotuberous ligaments. (Redrawn from Vleeming et al 1997.)

When the sacrum nutates relative to the innominate, a linear motion or translation between the two joint surfaces occurs. This is an arthrokinematic motion between two joint surfaces. The sacroiliac joint is shaped like a boomerang (Bowen & Cassidy 1981) with two arms at 90°. The short arm (S1) lies in a craniocaudal plane while the long arm (S2, 3, 4) lies in an anteroposterior plane. The two arms converge at the arcuate line of the innominate. In sacral nutation, the sacrum glides inferiorly down the short arm and posteriorly along the long arm (Fig. 5.8). This motion is resisted by the wedge shape of the sacrum, the ridges and depressions of the articular surface, the friction coefficient of the joint surface and the integrity of the interosseous and sacrotuberous ligaments (Vleeming et al 1990a,b). The ligaments are supported in this action by the muscles which insert into them (see kinetics section). The amplitude of this translation is extremely small (1–2 mm) and can be palpated (Ch. 7).

When the sacrum counternutates, the sacrum glides anteriorly along the long arm and superiorly up the short arm (Fig. 5.9). This

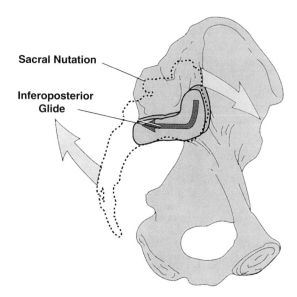

Figure 5.8 When the sacrum nutates, its articular surface glides inferoposteriorly relative to the innominate.

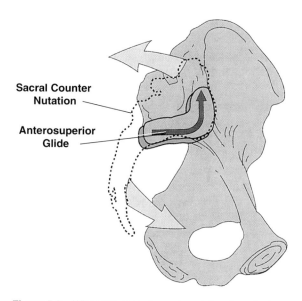

Figure 5.9 When the sacrum counternutates, its articular surface glides anterosuperiorly relative to the innominate.

motion is resisted by the long dorsal sacroiliac ligament (Fig. 4.15) (Vleeming et al 1996). This ligament is supported by the contraction of the multifidus which acts to nutate the sacrum. The multifidus and levator ani appear to act as a force couple to control sacral nutation/counter-nutation (Snijders et al 1997).

Anterior/posterior rotation of the innominate

Anterior rotation of the innominate occurs bilaterally during forward bending of the trunk and when rising to the seated position from supine lying. During this motion, there is no relative rotation between the innominates: the pelvic girdle is rotating as a unit forward on the femora. Unilateral anterior rotation of the innominate occurs during extension of the lower extremity. This motion does produce movement within the pelvic girdle itself and is the same as sacral counternutation.

Posterior rotation of the innominate occurs bilaterally during backward bending of the trunk. During this motion, there is no relative rotation between the innominates themselves, as the pelvic girdle is rotating as a unit backward on the femora. Unilateral posterior rotation occurs during flexion of the lower extremity. This motion does produce movement within the pelvic girdle itself and is the same as sacral nutation.

When the innominate anteriorly rotates, it glides inferiorly down the short arm and posteriorly along the long arm of the sacroiliac joint (Fig. 5.10). This is the same arthrokinematic motion as sacral counternutation. When the innominate posteriorly rotates, it glides anteriorly along the long arm and superiorly up the short arm (Fig. 5.11). This is the same arthrokinematic motion as sacral nutation.

Kinematics of the hip

The femur articulates with the innominate via a ball-and-socket joint, the hip, which is capable of circumductive motion. The hip is classified as an unmodified ovoid joint and in mechanical terms is capable of 12 degrees of freedom of motion along and about three perpendicular axes (Fig. 5.12). Again, this classification does not account for the anatomical factors which influence the coupling of motion which actually occurs at the joint.

Flexion/extension occurs when either the pelvic girdle as a unit or the free femur rotates about a coronal axis through the center of the femoral head and neck. Approximately 100° of

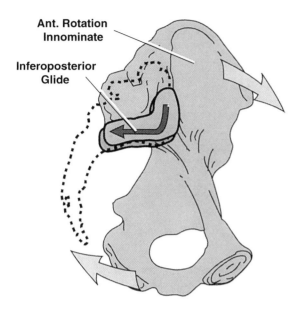

Figure 5.10 When the innominate anteriorly rotates, its articular surface glides inferoposteriorly relative to the sacrum.

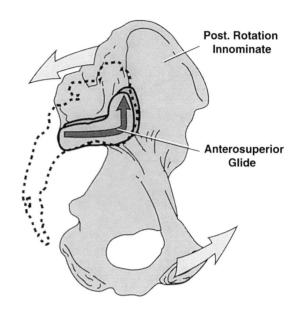

Figure 5.11 When the innominate posteriorly rotates, its articular surface glides anterosuperiorly relative to the sacrum.

femoral flexion is possible, following which motion of the sacroiliac and intervertebral joints occurs to allow the anterior thigh to approximate the chest (Warwick & Williams 1989). Approximately 20° of femoral extension is possible (Kapandji 1970). When rotation of the femoral head occurs purely about this axis (i.e. without conjoined abduction/adduction or medial/lateral rotation) the motion is described as a pure spin.

Abduction/adduction occurs when either the pelvic girdle as a unit or the free femur rotates about a sagittal axis through the center of the femoral head. Approximately 45° of femoral abduction and 30° of femoral adduction are possible, following which the pelvic girdle laterally bends beneath the vertebral column (Kapandji 1970). When the femur rotates purely about this sagittal axis, the head of the femur transcribes a superoinferior chord within the acetabulum (i.e. the shortest distance between two points); therefore this motion is described as a pure swing.

Medial/lateral rotation occurs when either the pelvic girdle as a unit or the free femur rotates about a longitudinal axis. The location of this axis is dependent upon fixation of the foot.

When the pelvic girdle rotates about a firmly planted foot, the longitudinal axis of rotation runs from the center of the femoral head through to the lateral femoral condyle. When the foot is off the ground, the femur can rotate about a variety of longitudinal axes all of which pass through the femoral head and the foot (Warwick & Williams 1989). Approximately 30° to 40° of medial rotation and 60° of lateral rotation are possible (Kapandji 1970). Pure femoral rotation about this axis causes the femoral head to transcribe an anteroposterior chord within the acetabulum and this motion is described as a pure swing.

Habitual movement of the femur relative to the innominate does not produce pure arthrokinematic motion. Rather, combinations of movement are the norm. The habitual pattern of motion for the non-weight-bearing lower extremity is a combination of flexion, abduction and lateral rotation and extension, adduction and medial rotation. Arthrokinematically, both motions are impure swings. During gait, the movement pattern consists of femoral flexion, adduction and lateral rotation, followed by extension, abduction and medial rotation which arthrokinematically are impure swings as well.

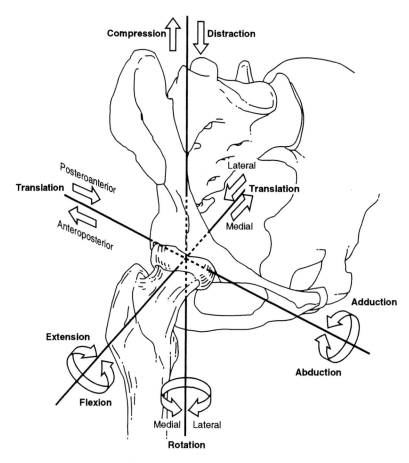

Figure 5.12 The osteokinematic motion of the femur. In mechanical terms, the femur is capable of 12 degrees of freedom of motion along and about three perpendicular axes.

KINETICS OF THE LUMBO-PELVIC-HIP REGION

The lumbo-pelvic-hip region is required to transmit the weight of the head, trunk and upper extremities to the lower extremities as well as to resist the forces incurred during motion of the upper and lower extremities. The mechanism by which these tasks are accomplished constitutes the kinetic function.

Panjabi (1992) has proposed a conceptual model which describes the interaction between the components which provide stability (Fig. 5.13). His model was directed to the spine; however it can be applied to the entire musculoskeletal system. In this model, he

describes three systems: passive, active and control. The passive system pertains to the osteoarticularligamentous structures, the active system pertains to the myofascia and the control system coordinates the actions of all. In addition, with respect to stability, Panjabi (1992) has defined a zone of motion which he has called the neutral zone (Fig. 5.14). This is a small range of displacement near the joint's neutral position where minimal resistance is given by the osteoligamentous structures. He has found that the range of the neutral zone may increase with injury, articular degeneration and/or weakness of the stabilizing musculature.

Snijders and Vleeming (Snijders et al 1993a,b, 1997, Vleeming et al 1990a,b, 1995b, 1997) have

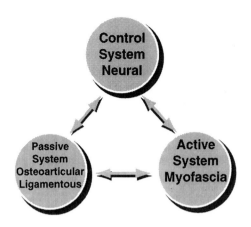

Figure 5.13   Conceptual model from Panjabi (1992) illustrating the components which provide stability.

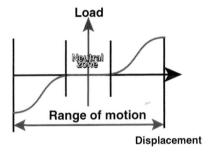

Figure 5.14   The neutral zone (Panjabi 1992) is a small range of displacement near the neutral joint position where minimal resistance is given by the osteoligamentous structures.

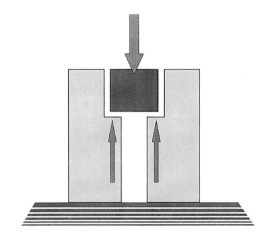

Figure 5.15   Schematic representation of form closure (Snijders et al 1993a).

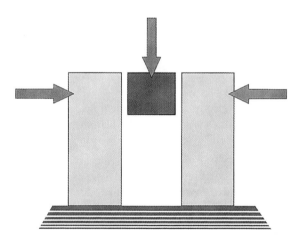

Figure 5.16   Schematic representation of force closure (Snijders et al 1993a).

used the terms form and force closure to describe the passive and active components of stability.

'Form closure refers to a stable situation with closely fitting joint surfaces, where no extra forces are needed to maintain the state of the system' (Snijders et al 1993a,b, 1997) (Fig. 5.15). The degree of inherent form closure of any joint depends on its anatomy. There are three factors which contribute to form closure; the shape of the joint surface, the friction coefficient of the articular cartilage and the integrity of the ligaments which approximate the joint.

'In the case of force closure, extra forces are needed to keep the object in place. Here friction must be present' (Snijders et al 1993a, 1997) (Fig. 5.16). Joints with predominantly flat surfaces are well suited to transfer large moments of force but

are vulnerable to shear. Factors which increase intra-articular compression will increase the friction coefficient and the ability of the joint to resist translation. Adequate compression through the joint must be the result of all forces acting across the joint if stability is to be insured and load transferred efficiently and safely.

Consequently, the stability of a system (the ability to effectively transfer load through joints) is dynamic and depends on many factors acting at the moment. These factors are both intrinsic and extrinsic to the system and include the following.

Intrinsic factors

- Osseous integrity.
- Articular/ligamentous integrity.
- Myofascial integrity which includes the:
  - ability of muscles to contract tonically in a sustained manner;
  - ability of the muscles to perform in a coordinated manner (motor control) such that the resultant force is adequate compression through the articular structures at an optimal point which controls the quantity of glide within the neutral zone.
- Neural (peripheral and central) control which ultimately orchestrates the appropriate motor control. This requires:
  - constant accurate afferent input from the mechanoreceptors in the joint and surrounding soft tissues;
  - appropriate interpretation of the afferent input and a suitable motor response

Extrinsic factors

- Gravity produces both vertical and horizontal shear forces which must be transferred through the system.

For every individual, there are many strategies available to achieve stability. These are based on the individual's intrinsic factors (i.e. connective tissue extensibility, muscle strength, body weight, joint surface shape) and the loads they need to control. When the load is increased (larger lever arm and/or weight) more compression or approximation of the articular surfaces is required for efficient load transfer.

Stability is not only about the quantity of motion (angular or linear) and the quality of the end feel, but about the control of systems which allow load to be transferred and movement to be smooth and effortless. When motor control is abnormal, there may be too much or too little approximation of the joint surfaces. In both cases, the resultant afferent input is distorted and sustains the abnormal motor control. The joint play tests (Ch. 7) for mobility and stability help to determine the quantity of compression present, both at rest and during contraction of muscles whose function is to control the neutral zone.

Chapter 9 will elaborate further on the specific findings of these tests as they relate to pathomechanical conditions of the sacroiliac joint.

The next sections will consider the components of the lumbar spine, pelvic girdle and hip which contribute to form and force closure and efficient load transfer through joints.

Kinetics of the lumbar spine

The kinetic analysis of the lumbar spine pertains to the study of the anatomical factors which resist the compression, torsion and postero-anterior shear which occur during the transference of loads from the trunk to the lower extremity and during activities of prehension of the upper extremity.

Compression

Compression of an object results when two forces act towards each other (see Fig. 5.1) The main restraint to compression in the lumbar spine is the vertebral body/annulus–nucleus unit, although the zygapophyseal joints have been noted (Bogduk 1997, Farfan 1973, Gracovetsky et al 1985, Gracovetsky & Farfan 1986, Kirkaldy-Willis 1983) to support up to 20% of the axial compression load (Fig. 5.17). Both the annulus and the nucleus transmit the load equally to the end-plate of the vertebral body. The thin cortical shell of the vertebral body provides the bulk of the compression strength, being simultaneously supported by a hydraulic mechanism within the cancellous core, the contribution of which is dependent upon the rate of loading. When compression is applied slowly (static loading), the nuclear pressure rises distributing its force onto the annulus and the end-plates. The annulus bulges circumferentially and the end-plates bow towards the vertebral bodies. Fluid is squeezed out of the cancellous core via the veins; however, when the rate of compression is increased, the small vessel size may retard the rate of outflow such that the internal pressure of the vertebral body rises, thus increasing the compressive strength of the unit. In this manner, the vertebral body supports and

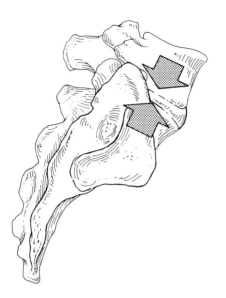

Figure 5.17 Compression of the lumbosacral junction.

protects the intervertebral disc against compression overload. The anatomical structure which initially yields to high loads of compression is the hyaline cartilage of the end-plate, suggesting that this structure is weaker than the peripheral parts of the end-plate (Bogduk 1997). The fracture appears radiographically as a Schmorl's node (Fig. 5.18) (Kirkaldy-Willis et al 1978, 1983). This lesion is commonly seen at the higher

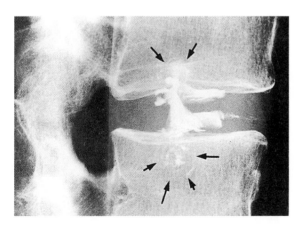

Figure 5.18 Superior and inferior end-plate fractures (Schmorl's nodes) detected via a discogram. Note the penetration of the dye into both the superior and inferior vertebral bodies through the end-plate (arrows). (Reproduced with permission from Farfan 1973.)

lumbar levels. The zygapophyseal joints do not contribute to weight bearing when in the neutral position, given that their sagittal and coronal components are oriented vertically. When the segment is extended, the inferior articular process of the superior vertebra glides inferiorly and impacts the pars interarticularis. When axial compression is applied in this lordotic position, load can be transferred through the inferior articular process to the lamina (Bogduk 1997).

When the thoracodorsal fascia is tight, the lumbar segments are under increased compressive loads during forward bending of the trunk. Over time, this can lead to multiple levels of minor disc protrusions, a finding which can be confirmed on CT scan. Treatment strategies which improve the flexibility of the thoracodorsal fascia will, in this instance, reduce the compressive loads through the lumbar spine.

Torsion

When a force is applied to an object at any location other than the center of rotation, it will cause the object to rotate about an axis through this pivot point. The magnitude of the torque force can be calculated by multiplying the quantity of the force by the distance the force acts from the pivot. Axial torsion of the lumbar vertebra occurs when the bone rotates about a vertical axis through the center of the body (Fig. 5.19) and is resisted by anatomical factors located within the vertebral arch (65%) as well as by the structures of the vertebral body/intervertebral disc unit (35%) (Bogduk 1997, Gracovetsky & Farfan 1986).

At the lumbosacral junction, the superior articular process of the sacrum (see Fig. 4.2) is squat and strong as opposed to the inferior articular process of the L5 vertebra which is much longer and receives less support from the pedicle. Consequently, the inferior process is more easily deflected when the zygapophyseal joint is loaded at 90° to its articular surface. This process can deflect 8° to 9° medially during axial torsion beyond which trabecular fractures and residual strain deformation will occur (Bogduk 1997, Farfan 1973).

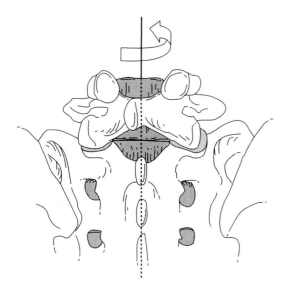

Figure 5.19 Right axial torsion of the L5 vertebra is resisted by osseous impaction of the left zygapophyseal joint and capsular distraction of the right zygapophyseal joint as well as by the segmental ligaments, the intervertebral disc and the myofascia.

The structure and orientation of the annular fibers is critical to the ability of the intervertebral disc to resist torsion. 'The concentric arrangement of the collagenous layers of the annulus ensures that when the disk is placed in tension, shear or rotation, the individual fibers are always in tension' (Kirkaldy-Willis 1983). Under static loading conditions, injuries occur with as little as 2° and certainly by 3.5° of axial rotation (Gracovetsky & Farfan 1986). The iliolumbar ligament (see Figs 4.12, 4.19) plays an important role in minimizing torque forces at the lumbosacral junction. The longer the transverse process of the L5 vertebra and consequently the shorter the iliolumbar ligament, the stronger is the resistance of the segment to torsion (Farfan 1973).

Axial compression also increases the segmental torque strength by 35% (Gracovetsky & Farfan 1986). During forward flexion of the lumbar spine, the instantaneous center of rotation moves forward (see Fig. 5.3) thus increasing the compressive load and consequently the ability of the joint to resist torsion (Farfan 1973, Gracovetsky & Farfan 1986).

Posteroanterior shear

Shear occurs when an applied force produces sliding between two planes (see Fig. 5.1). Posteroanterior shear occurs in the lumbar spine when a force attempts to displace a superior vertebra anterior to the one below (Fig. 5.20). The anatomical factors which resist posteroanterior shear at the lumbosacral junction are primarily the impaction of the inferior articular processes of L5 against the superior articular processes of the sacrum and the iliolumbar ligaments (Bogduk 1997). Secondary factors include the intervertebral disc, the anterior longitudinal ligament, the posterior longitudinal ligament and the midline posterior ligamentous system (Twomey & Taylor 1985).

Dynamically, the posterior midline ligaments, the thoracodorsal fascia and the muscles which generate tension within this system are important in balancing the anterior shear forces which occur when large loads are lifted (force closure) (Adams & Dolan 1997, Bogduk 1997, Gracovetsky & Farfan 1986, Hides et al 1994, 1996, Hodges & Richardson 1996, Richardson & Jull 1995, Vleeming et al 1990a,b, 1995a, 1997). The optimal method of loading the spine should balance both compression and shear such that the magnitude of the resultant force does not exceed the strength of the joint. Consequently,

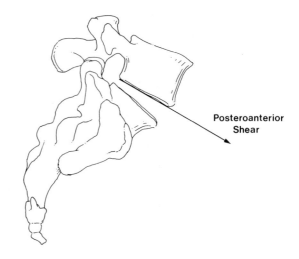

Posteroanterior Shear

Figure 5.20 Posteroanterior shear of the L5 vertebra on the sacrum.

both the articular (form closure) and the myofascial components (force closure) are required to balance the moment of a large external load.

We have found that for any load, for minimum equalized stress, there is a privileged stable zone corresponding to the situation in which the moment will be balanced and shared in equal thirds by muscle, midline ligament system, and by the abdominals through the thoracolumbar fascia (Gracovetsky & Farfan 1986).

The thoracodorsal fascia is supported by the contraction of the transversus abdominis and the multifidus muscles. Recent research (Hodges & Richardson 1996, 1997a, Richardson & Jull 1995), has shown that the transversus abdominis is a primary muscle for stabilization of the lumbar spine. It has a large attachment to the middle layer and the deep lamina of the posterior layer of the thoracodorsal fascia (Fig. 4.33) and is recruited *prior* to the initiation of any movement of the upper or lower extremity (Hodges & Richardson 1996). In this study of patients with chronic low back pain, a timing delay was found in which the transversus abdominis muscle failed to contract prior to the initiation of arm and/or leg motion. Hodges & Richardson conclude that:

a significant motor control deficit is present in people with chronic low back pain which is primarily associated with the control of contraction of transversus abdominis. The failure of the stabilization mechanism with subjects in the LBP [low back pain] group indicates that the normal strategy used by the body to control intervertebral motion and stiffness is inefficient.

In a separate study, Hides et al (1994) found wasting and local inhibition at a segmental level of the lumbar multifidus muscle in all patients with a first episode of acute/subacute low back pain. In a follow-up study (Hides et al 1996), they found that without therapeutic intervention, the multifidus did not regain its original size or function and the recurrence rate of low back pain over an 8-month period was very high. They also found that the deficit could be reversed with an appropriate exercise program.

The thoracodorsal fascia and its supporting musculature bridge the lumbar spine and pelvic

girdle (Fig. 4.20). While it plays a significant role in stabilization of the lumbar spine, it is also significant in the transference of force from the trunk to the lower extremity (Vleeming et al 1995a). The role of the transversus abdominis and multifidus will be further discussed in the section on the kinetics of the pelvic girdle, below.

Kinetics of the pelvic girdle

The kinetic analysis of the pelvic girdle pertains to the study of the anatomical factors which maintain the integrity of the pelvic girdle and resist the translation forces which occur during the transference of loads from the trunk to the lower extremity and during activities of prehension of the upper extremity.

The pelvic girdle demonstrates a self-locking mechanism (Snidjers et al 1993a,b, 1997, Vleeming et al 1990a,b, 1997) which incorporates both form and force closure. With respect to form closure, the shape of the sacroiliac joint is highly variable both between and within individuals (Fig. 3.6). In the skeletally mature, S1, S2 and S3 contribute to the formation of the sacral surface and each part can be oriented in a different vertical plane (Fig 4.2). In addition, the sacrum is wedged anteroposteriorly. These factors provide resistance to both vertical and horizontal translation. In the young, the wedging is incomplete, such that the sacroiliac joint is planar at all three levels and is vulnerable to shear forces until ossification is complete (third decade).

The articular cartilage lining the sacroiliac joint is unusual. The sacral surface is lined with smooth hyaline cartilage whereas the iliac surface is lined with a rough type of fibro-cartilage. Vleeming et al (1990b) studied the friction coefficient of the sacroiliac joint and found that the coarse cartilage texture contributed to the ability of the joint to resist translation. The coarseness of the iliac cartilage increases with age (Bowen & Cassidy 1981). The complementary ridges and grooves in the mature sacroiliac joint (Solonen 1957, Vleeming et al 1990b) also increase friction and thus contribute to form closure.

The sacroiliac joint is surrounded by some of the strongest ligaments in the body. The long dorsal sacroiliac ligament tightens during sacral counternutation or anterior rotation of the innominate (Vleeming et al 1996) (Fig. 4.15). The sacrotuberous and interosseous ligaments tighten during sacral nutation or posterior rotation of the innominate (Fig. 5.7) (Vleeming et al 1989a,b, Vleeming et al 1997). Vleeming et al (1997) found that when the sacrum moves toward nutation the increase in the ligamentous tension facilitates the force closure mechanism thus increasing compression through the sacro-iliac joint. Compression of articular structures is essential for efficient load transfer; therefore, sacral nutation is more stable than counter-nutation. The ventral sacroiliac ligaments are the weakest of the group and are supported anteriorly by the integrity of the pubic symphysis.

When considering the muscles which contri-bute to stability of the pelvic girdle (and the lumbar spine and hip), there are two important groups: the inner unit and the outer unit. The inner unit consists of the muscles of the pelvic floor, transversus abdominis, multifidus and the diaphragm (Fig. 5.21). The outer unit consists of four systems: the posterior oblique (Fig. 5.22), the deep longitudinal (Fig. 5.23), the anterior oblique (Fig. 5.24) and the lateral (Fig. 5.25).

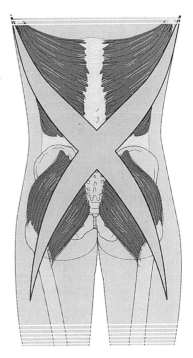

Figure 5.22 The posterior oblique system of the outer unit includes the latissimus dorsi, gluteus maximus and the intervening thoracodorsal fascia. (Redrawn from Vleeming et al 1995a.)

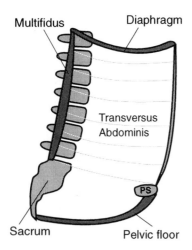

Figure 5.21 The muscles of the inner unit include the multifidus, transversus abdominis, diaphragm and the pelvic floor.

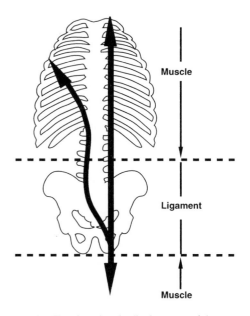

Figure 5.23 The deep longitudinal system of the outer unit consists of erector spinae, the deep lamina of the thoracodorsal fascia, the sacrotuberous ligament and the biceps femoris muscle. (Redrawn from Gracovetsky 1997.)

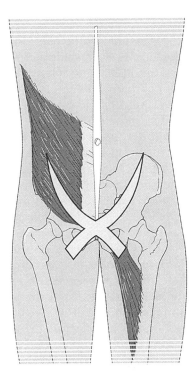

Figure 5.24 The anterior oblique system of the outer unit includes the external and internal oblique, the contralateral adductors of the thigh and the intervening anterior abdominal fascia.

The inner unit

The function of the four parts of the levator ani muscle and the inter-relationship between the pelvic floor and the abdominals has received recent study (Sapsford et al 1998). Using fine-needle insertion electromyography (EMG) into the pubococcygeus and the abdominals, they found that activation of the abdominal muscles is a normal response to contraction of the pelvic floor. When the abdominal muscles were recruited strongly, the entire pelvic floor contracted in response. When the individual abdominal muscles were selectively recruited gently, the pelvic floor responded with a specific response. Although the research is not complete, the hypothesis is that pubococcygeus tends to contract with transversus abdominis, and iliococcygeus and ischiococcygeus with the oblique abdominals. Rectus abdominis is thought to be associated with puborectalis.

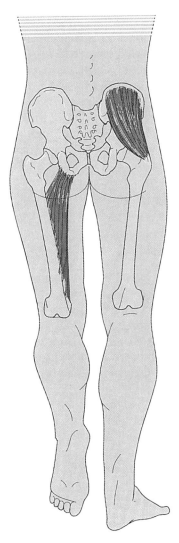

Figure 5.25 The lateral system of the outer unit includes the gluteus medius and minimus and the contralateral adductors of the thigh.

Sapsford specializes in the treatment of urinary and anorectal dysfunction and has found that patients are able to isolate the muscles of the pelvic floor more effectively when their abdominal wall is incorporated into the training. Contraction of the iliococcygeus and ischiococcygeus bilaterally will counternutate the sacrum; the multifidus will nutate the sacrum. Together, the levator ani and multifidus act as a force couple to control the position of the sacrum. When the sacrum is held secure by these two muscles, the base of the spine is more stable. The transversus abdominis has been previously discussed in terms of its role in stabilization of the lumbar spine. Contraction of this muscle increases the tension laterally in the thoracodorsal fascia and helps to increase the intra-abdominal pressure (Hodges & Richardson 1996, Vleeming et al 1997). When acting in conjunction with the muscles of the outer unit, contraction of the transversus abdominis can increase the tension in the posterior sacroiliac ligaments through the thoracodorsal fascia, and thus augment the force closure mechanism.

The outer unit

There are four systems which comprise the outer unit: the posterior oblique, the deep longitudinal, the anterior oblique and the lateral. The posterior oblique system (Fig. 5.22) includes the latissimus dorsi, gluteus maximus and the intervening thoracodorsal fascia. The fibers of the gluteus maximus muscle run perpendicular to the plane of the sacroiliac joint and blend with the thoracodorsal fascia and the contralateral latissimus dorsi (Vleeming et al 1995a) (Fig. 4.20). Compression of the sacroiliac joint occurs when the gluteus maximus and the contralateral latissimus dorsi contract. This compression approximates the posterior aspect of the innominates (Snijders et al 1997, Vleeming et al 1995a, 1997) and contributes to the force closure mechanism. This oblique system is a significant contributor to load transference through the pelvic girdle during rotational activities (Mooney 1997) and during gait (Gracovetsky 1997, Greenman 1997, Vleeming et al 1997).

The deep longitudinal system (Fig. 5.23) includes the erector spinae muscle, the deep lamina of the thoracodorsal fascia, the sacrotuberous ligament and the biceps femoris muscle (Gracovetsky 1997, Vleeming et al 1997). This system can also increase tension in the thoracodorsal fascia and facilitate compression through the sacroiliac joints. In addition, the biceps femoris can control the degree of sacral nutation through its connections to the sacrotuberous ligament (Wingerden et al 1993).

The anterior oblique system (Fig. 5.24) includes the oblique abdominals, the contralateral adductor muscles (Snijders et al 1995) of the thigh and the intervening anterior abdominal fascia. The oblique abdominals are thought (Richardson & Jull 1995) to be primarily phasic muscles which initiate movement, and prior contraction of the transversus abdominis is required for stabilization of the trunk (Hodges & Richardson 1996). They are involved in all activities of the trunk and upper and lower extremities. While they remain active in unsupported sitting, Snijders et al (1995, 1997) found that they become quiet when the legs are crossed. They propose that the tension generated through the passive structures of the lumbo-pelvic-hip region when sitting cross-legged is sufficient to stabilize the pelvic girdle and the force closure mechanism is not needed. They have observed that seated individuals vary their posture frequently and propose that one alternates between a passive method of stabilization and an active one to conserve energy and reduce passive strain.

The lateral system (Fig. 5.25) includes the gluteus medius and minimus and the contralateral adductors of the thigh. Although these muscles are not directly involved in force closure of the sacroiliac joint, they are significant for the function of the pelvic girdle during standing and walking and are reflexively inhibited when the sacroiliac joint is unstable.

Weakness, or insufficient recruitment and/or timing, of the muscles of the inner and/or outer unit reduces the force closure mechanism through the sacroiliac joint. The patient then adopts compensatory movement strategies (Lee 1997a) to accommodate the weakness. This can lead to decompensation of the lower back, hip and knee.

Kinetics of the hip

The hip is subjected to forces equal to multiples of the body weight and requires osseous, articular and myofascial integrity for stability. The factors which contribute to stability at the hip include the anatomical configuration of the joint as well as the orientation of the trabeculae, the strength and orientation of the capsule and the ligaments during habitual movements, and the strength of the periarticular muscles and fascia.

During erect standing, the superincumbent body weight is distributed equally through the pelvic girdle to the femoral heads and necks. Each hip joint supports approximately 33% of the body weight which subsequently produces a bending moment between the neck of the femur and its shaft (Singleton & LeVeau 1975). A complex system of bony trabeculae exists within the femoral head and neck to prevent supero-inferior shearing of the femoral head during erect standing (Fig. 5.26) (Kapandji 1970).

The orientation of the capsule and the articular ligaments (see Figs 4.28, 4.29) also contributes to stability at the hip during habitual motion (Table 5.2). Extension of the femur winds all of the

extra-articular ligaments around the femoral neck and renders them taut. The inferior band of the iliofemoral ligament is under the greatest tension in extension. Flexion of the femur unwinds the extra-articular ligaments, and when combined with slight adduction, predisposes the femoral head to posterior dislocation if sufficient force is applied to the distal end of the femur (e.g. dashboard impact).

During lateral rotation of the femur, the iliotrochanteric band of the iliofemoral ligament and the pubofemoral ligament become taut while the ischiofemoral ligament becomes slack. Conversely, during medial rotation of the femur, the anterior ligaments become slack while the ischiofemoral ligament becomes taut.

Abduction of the femur tenses the pubo-femoral ligament, and the inferior band of the iliofemoral ligament as well as the ischiofemoral ligament. At the end of abduction, the neck of the femur impacts onto the acetabular rim, thus distorting and everting the labrum (Kapandji 1970). In this manner, the acetabular labrum deepens the articular cavity (improving form closure) thus increasing stability without limiting mobility. Adduction results in tension of the iliotrochanteric band of the iliofemoral

Body weight

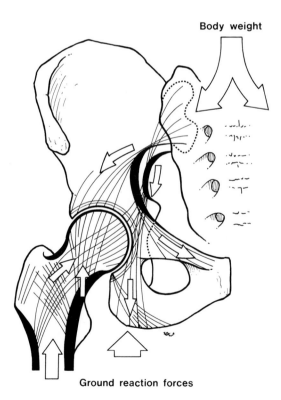

Ground reaction forces

Figure 5.26 The orientation of the bony trabeculae within the pelvic girdle corresponds to the lines of force met in both static and dynamic function. (Redrawn from Kapandji 1970.)

Table 5.2 Resultant tension of the extra-articular ligaments of the hip joint during motion of the femur

Femoral motion	Ligament	Tension
Extension	All extra-articular ligaments	Taut
Flexion/adduction	All ligaments	Slack
Lateral rotation	Iliotrochanteric	Taut
	Pubofemoral	Taut
	Ischiofemoral	Slack
Medial rotation	Iliofemoral	Slack
	Pubofemoral	Slack
	Ischiofemoral	Taut
Abduction	Pubofemoral	Taut
	Inferior band*	Taut
	Ischiofemoral	Taut
	Iliotrochanteric	Slack
Adduction	Iliotrochanteric	Taut
	Inferior band*	Slack
	Ischiofemoral	Slack
	Pubofemoral	Slack

*Inferior band of iliofemoral ligament.

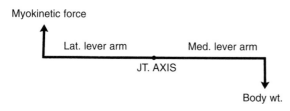

MYOKINETIC FORCE × LATERAL LEVER ARM
= BODY WEIGHT × MEDIAL LEVER ARM

Figure 5.27 The kinetic forces medial and lateral to the axis of the hip joint must be equal if balance is to be preserved.

ligament while the others remain relatively slack.

The ligamentum teres is under moderate tension in erect standing as well as during medial and lateral rotation of the femur. Kapandji (1970) notes that the acetabular fossa outlines the extreme positions of the foveal attachment of the ligamentum teres during habitual motion.

The passive system receives dynamic support from the multiple muscles which cross and also attach to the capsule of the hip joint. Standing on one limb dramatically increases the magnitude of forces which must be met at the hip joint (2.4 to 2.6 times the body weight) and subsequently requires recruitment of the periarticular muscles for maintenance of equilibrium. The body weight must be shifted such that the line of gravity falls through the supporting limb distally. The force developed by the muscle contraction, multiplied by the length of the lateral lever arm to the joint axis, must be balanced by the force developed by the body weight, multiplied by the length of the medial lever arm to the joint axis, if balance is to be preserved (Fig. 5.27). Consequently, one-legged stance can be a useful clinical test of kinetic function of the hip joint. The longer the lever arm, the more articular compression needed for stability.

FUNCTIONAL BIOMECHANICS

The integrated biomechanics of the lumbo-pelvic-hip region during functional movements need to be understood, since these are the motions that are evaluated in the clinic. Since the specific biomechanics of each region have been described, a more integrated perspective can now be discussed.

Forward bending of the trunk results in a posterior displacement of the pelvic girdle as a unit which shifts the center of gravity behind the pedal base (Figs 5.28, 5.29). The innominates anteriorly rotate bilaterally on the femoral heads about a transverse axis through the hip joints. The lumbar spine forward bends in a supero-inferior direction until L5 flexes and anteriorly translates on the sacrum.

Within the pelvic girdle itself, there is no relative anteroposterior rotation between the innominates during forward bending. Both PSISs of the innominates should travel an equal distance in a superior direction as the pelvic girdle flexes on the femoral heads. There is a slight outward rotation of both innominates which can be felt as an approximation of the PSISs (Vleeming et al 1997). In standing, the sacrum rests in slight nutation (Sturesson et al 1989). This nutation can be felt to increase in some during the first 60° of forward bending. Once the extensibility of the deep longitudinal system (biceps femoris, sacrotuberous ligament and the deep lamina of the posterior layer of the thoracodorsal fascia) has been reached, the relative flexibility of the sacrum becomes less than the innominates. The innominates then continue to anteriorly rotate on the femoral heads (flexion at the hip joint) resulting in a relative counternutation of the sacrum. The stage at which this reversal of sacral motion occurs appears to be critical to stability of the sacroiliac joint. Sacral nutation facilitates compression and thus stability for the sacroiliac joint, whereas counternutation is the position of vulnerability (Vleeming et al 1997). If the sacrum remains nutated throughout forward bending, the sacroiliac joint remains compressed and loads can be more effectively transferred through the pelvic girdle to the lower extremity. When the sacrum counternutates early, as in individuals with very tight hamstrings, the sacroiliac joint is less compressed and more motor control is required for load transference. Many low back injuries occur in this position.

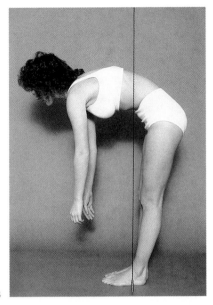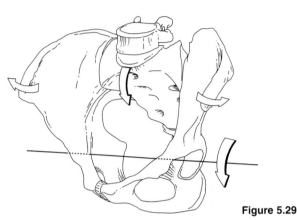

Figure 5.28 **Figure 5.29**

Figures 5.28 and 5.29   Forward bending of the trunk from the erect standing position, and the osteokinematic motion of the pelvic girdle.

In summary, in some, nutation persists throughout forward bending. In others, a slight counternutation (unlocking) occurs towards the end of the range. This is not thought to be normal (Vleeming, personal communication).

It has been shown (Basmajian & Deluca 1985) that among the mammals, man has the most efficient posture in bipedal stance. In the lumbo-pelvic-hip region intermittent bursts of activity from the gluteus medius, tensor fascia lata and the hamstring muscles are required to control postural sway. Constant activity has been reported (Basmajian & Deluca 1985) in the iliopsoas muscle to support the iliofemoral ligament of the hip joint, as well as in the internal oblique muscle to protect the inguinal canal. All other muscle groups are quiescent when standing is optimal. Deviation from this economical position results in the immediate recruitment of both the trunk and femoral musculature, thus dramatically increasing the energy expenditure of standing still.

The muscles which eccentrically control forward bending of the trunk and the pelvic girdle include the erector spinae, multifidus, quadratus lumborum and the hip joint extensors (gluteus maximus and the hamstrings). Contributions from the hip joint rotators, abductors and adductors as well as from the deep back muscles function to stabilize and coordinate the motion between the lumbar spine, pelvic girdle and hip. Prior to this motion, stabilization of the lumbar segments and the sacrum is required from the inner unit of muscles, in particular, the transversus abdominis, multifidus and the pelvic floor.

Backward bending of the trunk (Figs 5.30, 5.31) results in an anterior displacement of the pelvic girdle and a shift of the center of gravity anterior to the pedal base. The thoracolumbar spine extends in a superoinferior direction until L5 extends and posteriorly translates on the sacrum. Within the pelvic girdle itself, there is no anteroposterior rotation between the two innominates as the pelvic girdle extends at the hip joint. Both PSISs should travel an equal distance in an inferior direction as the unit extends on the femoral heads. The sacrum should remain in its nutated position relative to the innominates.

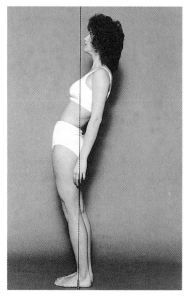

Figure 5.30

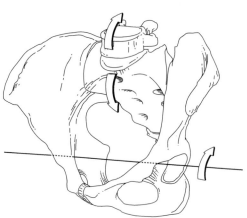

Figure 5.31

Figures 5.30 and 5.31   Backward bending of the trunk from the erect standing position, and the osteokinematic motion of the pelvic girdle.

The muscles which eccentrically control backward bending of the trunk include the abdominals, the quadriceps, the tensor fascia lata (anterior component) and the iliopsoas. Contributions from the hip joint rotators, abductors and adductors as well as the deep back muscles function to stabilize and coordinate the motion between the lumbar spine, pelvic girdle and hip. Prior to this motion, stabilization of the lumbar segments and the sacrum is required from the inner unit of muscles, in particular the transversus abdominis, multifidus and the pelvic floor.

During climbing or walking, a twist or torsion is produced within the pelvic girdle (Fig. 5.32). In the standing position, when the right femur is flexed, the right innominate posteriorly rotates and the sacrum rotates to the right. When the right femur is extended, the right innominate anteriorly rotates and the sacrum rotates to the left. When the pelvic girdle is twisted such that the right innominate posteriorly rotates, the left innominate anteriorly rotates and the sacrum rotates to the right, the right side of the sacrum is nutated and the left side is counternutated relative to the innominates.

The transference of body weight from a bipedal to unipedal stance requires coordinated facilitation and inhibition of specific muscle groups which are functions of the articular reflexes (i.e. input from the mechanoreceptors).

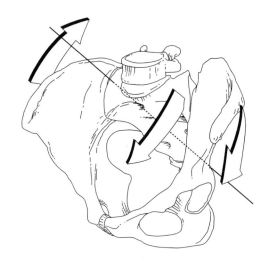

Figure 5.32   Right intra-pelvic torsion: posterior rotation of the right innominate, anterior rotation of the left innominate, right rotation of the sacrum (relative to the coronal body plane). This motion produces nutation at the right sacroiliac joint and counternutation at the left.

Unipedal stance requires stabilization of the pelvic girdle in the coronal plane and consequently the ipsilateral gluteus medius/minimus and tensor fascia lata muscles should be immediately facilitated. This facilitation occurs reflexively via the mechanoreceptors located in the ligamentum teres, which fire subsequent to compression of the femoral head into the acetabular fossa (Dee 1969). Standing on one leg and lifting the other requires effective form and force closure of the lumbo-pelvic-hip region. Loss of form closure (articular instability) on the weight-bearing side or force closure (myofascial weakness or incoordination of the inner and/or outer units) throughout the entire system is manifested readily during this motion.

Left lateral bending of the trunk while standing is initiated by displacing the upper legs to the right, thus maintaining the line of gravity central within the pedal base (Fig. 5.33). The apex of this lateral bending curve should be at the level of the greater trochanter. The pelvic girdle laterally bends to the left, as a unit, and rotates slightly to the right on the femoral heads. Minimal motion occurs within the pelvic girdle, although in the young, a slight twist can occur

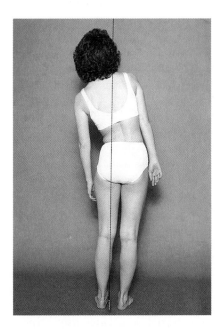

Figure 5.33 Left lateral bending of the trunk.

with the right innominate rotating posteriorly and the left anteriorly. In this instance, the sacrum rotates to the right relative to the coronal body plane. The right hip adducts and internally rotates, the left hip abducts and externally rotates. The lumbar spine laterally bends to the left. The segmental conjunct rotation is variable. Clinically, L5 appears to rotate/sideflex congruently with the sacrum.

The muscles which eccentrically control lateral bending of the trunk include the contralateral abdominals, erector spinae, multifidus, quadratus lumborum, iliacus, psoas, piriformis, tensor fascia lata, gluteus medius, gluteus minimus and the ipsilateral adductors of the hip. Contributions from the hip joint rotators as well as the deep back muscles function to stabilize and coordinate the motion between the lumbar spine, pelvic girdle and hip.

Axial rotation of the pelvic girdle, together with axial rotation of the vertebral column, knees and feet, allows the eyes to scan 360° from a stationary point. During left axial rotation, the femora twist to the left about a midline vertical axis, resulting in an anteromedial displacement of the proximal right femur and a posteromedial displacement of the proximal left femur. Simultaneously, the pelvic girdle as a unit rotates to the left on the displaced femoral heads, resulting in extension and lateral rotation of the right femur and flexion and medial rotation of the left femur. The twist continues in an inferosuperior direction, producing intra-pelvic torsion. The right innominate anteriorly rotates while the left innominate posteriorly rotates. Both bones passively drive the sacrum into left rotation. The sacrum counternutates at the right sacroiliac joint and nutates at the left. The lumbar spine rotates to the left, the segmental conjunct rotation is variable. Clinically, L5 appears to rotate/sideflex congruently with the sacrum.

PREGNANCY

The pelvic girdle has been shown (Brooke 1930, Hagen 1974, Kristiansson 1997, Young 1940) to exhibit excessive mobility secondary to relaxation of the ligaments of the sacroiliac joints and the pubic symphysis during pregnancy. This process begins during the 4th month and continues until the 7th month of pregnancy, following which only a slight increase in mobility occurs. Great variation in the degree of both transverse and superoinferior widening of the pubic symphysis has been noted radiologically (Brooke 1930, Hagen 1952), with the average increase being 5 mm. A correlation between widening of the pubic symphysis and pelvic pain during pregnancy has not been found (Ostgaard 1997).

According to Hagen (1952), relaxation of the pelvic girdle in pregnancy is due to the presence of a specific high-molecular-weight hormone, relaxin, which together with oestrogen causes

... depolymerization of hyaluronic acid ...
Compressive, shearing and tensile forces constitute a chronic trauma increasing the concentration of hyaluronidase ... This interferes with the humoral conditions needed for pelvic stability and very likely also plays a certain role as a pathogenetic factor in pelvic relaxation.

This was recently confirmed by Kristiansson (1997).

Consequently, the locking mechanism of the pelvic girdle is less effective, thus increasing the strain on the ligaments of both the sacroiliac joints and the pubic symphysis. The morphological changes within the pelvic girdle associated with pregnancy are universal and often occur without symptoms. Occasionally, women present between the 26th and 28th weeks with increasing tenderness over the sacroiliac joint and/or pubic symphysis secondary to loss of kinetic function. Normally, the pelvic girdle returns to its pre-pregnant state between the 3rd and 6th months postpartum and simply requires external stabilization during this period (see Ch. 9).

In Europe, there is an increasing incidence of women who experience peripartum pelvic pain of an incapacitating nature (Heiberg & Aarseth 1997, Mens et al 1996, Ostgaard 1997). The pain develops during pregnancy and/or delivery and stability is not recovered within the normal time limits. Exercise programs similar to the one presented in this text are being used together with behavioral therapy with excellent functional outcomes (Vleeming, Spine and Joint Centre, Rotterdam, personal communication). The results from this program will be presented at the Third World Congress on Low Back Pain in Vienna, November 19–21, 1998.

LIFTING

Incorrect lifting technique is often responsible for the acute onset of pain in the lumbo-pelvic-hip region. Consequently, education with respect to 'safe' lifting methods is paramount to the rehabilitative process (see Ch. 11).

Moving an object from the floor to a higher surface initially requires forward bending of the trunk. Flexion of the spine is controlled by the eccentric contraction of the spinal extensors. Once the trunk is inclined 45° forward, the posterior ligamentous system and the thoraco-dorsal fascia become taut and the contraction of the spinal extensors ceases (Fig. 5.34) (Farfan 1973). The tension of the thoracodorsal fascia increases the force closure mechanism through the sacroiliac joints. At this point, the sacrum is nutated and the interosseous and sacrotuberous ligaments are taut. The ligamentous tension is supported by the muscles of the pelvic floor and the biceps femoris muscle. Subsequently, forward bending of the entire pelvic girdle occurs on the femoral heads (hip joint flexion).

When the spine is not under additional load (i.e. no weight in the arms) the sequence of forward bending can be varied at will such that forward bending of the pelvic girdle may occur prior to spinal flexion (Fig. 5.35). In this instance, continued isometric contraction of the thoraco-lumbar spinal extensors is required well beyond 45° of anterior inclination of the trunk since the posterior ligamentous system remains slack and therefore ineffectual in supporting a load. This movement pattern is commonly seen amongst dancers and in aerobics classes and if repeated often enough can become the individual's habitual movement pattern for forward bending.

As the external load increases, this altered movement pattern becomes less desirable since muscles are required to perform functions for which they are not ideally suited (Adams & Dolan 1997, Farfan 1975). 'When the weight-lifting strategy is changed from ligament to muscle, compression is increased for large angles of flexion. The ideal must be the use of ligament whenever possible, and this can best be done by maintaining the spine in flexion' (Gracovetsky & Farfan 1986).

The moment of the external load is reduced if the distance between the lifted object and the vertebral column is shortened. Thus, a flexible spine has the mechanical advantage of reducing the distance between the shoulders and the hips, hence decreasing the external load (Adams & Dolan 1997).

Returning to erect standing is initiated by backward rotation of the pelvis. This motion is produced by the concentric contraction of the gluteus maximus (Fig. 5.36). Load transference through the trunk is maintained by a coordinated action of the abdominals and deep spinal stabilizers. The sacroiliac joints are compressed and stability is maintained through the force closure mechanism provided by the tension in the thoracodorsal fascia caused by contraction of the latissimus dorsi, the transversus abdominis, multifidus and gluteus maximus. The gluteus maximus muscle has a considerable mechanical advantage in man as compared to other primates, given the increased anteroposterior depth of man's pelvis. In addition, more than half of the muscle inserts into the iliotibial band distally which increases its leverage on the hip joint, especially when the band is taut. The size and anatomy of this muscle render it an excellent 'lifter'.

As the trunk resumes its erect posture, the thoracolumbar spine begins to extend via concentric activity of the spinal extensors (Fig. 5.37). Clinically, this is a vulnerable point in the lift and a time when injuries often occur. The spinal musculature remains active until the load is released and erect stance is obtained.

There are two additional mechanisms which can assist in lifts of heavy loads. Both mechanisms rely on the thoracodorsal fascia and its attachments for their effect. The first involves an isometric contraction of the spinal extensor muscles at the beginning of the actual lift. The second involves an isometric contraction of the abdominal muscles throughout the lift.

The multifidus and the erector spinae muscles are contained within an envelope of the thoracodorsal fascia. The fascia is rendered taut when the muscles broaden as a consequence of their contraction (Fig. 4.33). This action decreases the anterior shear force at the L4 and L5 vertebrae via the midline fascial attachment to the spinous processes. More directly, the posteroanterior orientation of the lumbar iliocostalis and the lumbar longissimus muscles (see Figs 4.30, 4.31) at the L4 and L5 levels counteracts the detrimental anterior shear force when recruited isometrically.

The transversus abdominis and the internal oblique muscles facilitate the role of the thoracodorsal fascia in lifting by increasing the tension of the lateral border. When the lumbar spine is loaded in positions other than spinal flexion (i.e. between 0° and 40° of forward bending), the midline ligament and the posterior ligamentous system can still be utilized to counteract anterior shear if the lateral border of the thoracodorsal fascia is rendered taut via contraction of the transversus abdominis and the internal oblique muscles (Gracovetsky et al 1981).

In summary, optimal and therefore safe loading and unloading of the lumbo-pelvic-hip region during activities of daily living can only occur when the myokinematics and myokinetics subserve the kinetic and kinematic requirements of the bones and joints they stabilize and move. The coordinated muscle response depends on complex peripheral and central feedback and feedforward mechanisms (Hodges 1997b) which integrate the osseous, articular and muscular function.

GAIT

Efficient gait requires simultaneous displacement of the femora, innominates, sacrum and lumbar vertebrae in all three body planes, the sagittal, coronal and transverse. Although each

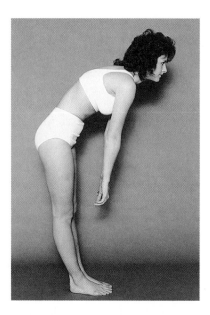

Figure 5.34 At 45° of forward bending, the posterior ligamentous system becomes taut and the eccentric activity of the spinal extensor muscles ceases.

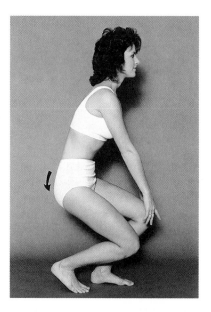

Figure 5.36 The concentric contraction of the hip extensor muscles rotates the pelvic girdle posteriorly. The co-contraction of the inner and outer units of muscles maintains lumbo-pelvic stability.

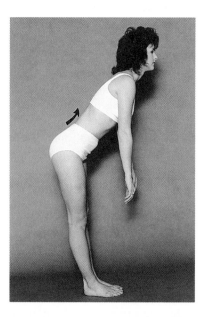

Figure 5.35 This movement pattern for forward bending (i.e. anterior rotation of the pelvic girdle prior to spinal flexion) is commonly seen amongst dancers and in aerobics classes.

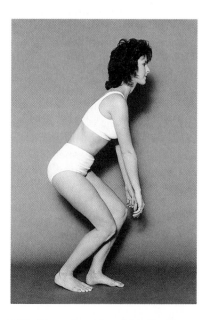

Figure 5.37 The vulnerable point in the lift occurs when the thoracolumbar spine begins to extend via the concentric activity of the spinal extensors.

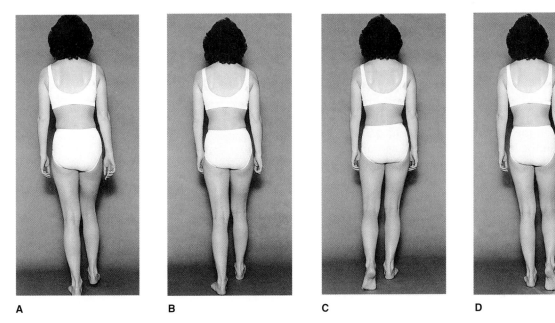

A   B   C   D

Figure 5.38   Gait. This sequence shows the right leg in swing phase, heel-strike, midstance and push-off, respectively.

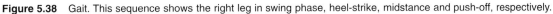

individual has his or her own pattern of walking (Fig. 5.38), the mandatory biomechanical requirements will be found in each. Walking is often an activity which magnifies symptoms when pathomechanics of the lumbo-pelvic-hip region are present. The following section will briefly outline the requirements of the lumbo-pelvic-hip region during one cycle of gait.

Femur

During the swing phase, the femur moves from an extended to a flexed position. The habitual movement pattern is not a pure spin at the hip joint but rather an arcuate (impure) swing and therefore conjoined osteokinematic motions also occur. During femoral flexion, adduction and lateral rotation occur. The capsular ligaments of the hip joint are taken from a maximum taut position in extension, abduction and medial rotation (i.e. the close pack position) to one of relatively loose pack in flexion, adduction and lateral rotation.

During the stance phase, the femur moves from a flexed to an extended position. Again, this motion is not a pure spin at the hip joint but

rather an arcuate or impure swing. The conjoined motions include abduction and medial rotation. The capsular ligaments are progressively wound around the femoral neck as the body weight passes anterior to the hip joint. Through the midstance position, the winding of the capsular ligaments of the hip joint, together with the osteokinetic and myokinetic forces, increases the compression of the femoral head into the acetabular fossa. Consequently, the mechanoreceptors in the ligamentum teres fire and reflexively facilitate the ipsilateral hip abductors. These muscles are necessary for stabilization of the pelvic girdle (lateral system).

Restrictions of femoral mobility may be the result of either hip joint restrictions or tight muscles and are manifested by a shortened stride length.

Pelvic girdle

During the swing phase, the pelvic girdle rotates, as a unit, on the femoral heads in the transverse plane towards the weight-bearing limb. The axis of this rotation is vertical between the two extremities and is dynamic rather than static. This motion decreases the amount of hip flexion/extension required for optimal stride length. Simultaneously, the pelvic girdle as a unit adducts on the weight-bearing limb, thus depressing the summit of the vertical rise of the center of gravity. Furthermore, intra-pelvic torsion in the sagittal plane (see Fig. 5.32) occurs between the innominates and the sacrum. Using the right extremity as an example, the pelvic girdle as a unit rotates transversely to the left, translates anteriorly and adducts on the left femoral head. Simultaneously, the right innominate posteriorly rotates and the left innominate anteriorly rotates driving the sacrum into right rotation. The sacrum nutates at the right sacroiliac joint and counternutates at the left (Greenman 1990, 1997). Posterior rotation of the innominate (right sacral nutation) increases the tension of the sacrotuberous and interosseous ligament and prepares the joint for heel strike (Fig. 5.39). The increase in tension contributes to the force closure mechanism, augments the form closure mechanism and therefore increases compression through the sacroiliac joint and thus its stability.

Inman et al (1981) have shown that the hamstrings become active just before heel strike. Contraction of the biceps femoris muscle increases the tension in the sacrotuberous ligament, further contributing to the force closure mechanism.

During the right single-leg stance phase, the pelvic girdle as a unit rotates to the right, translates anteriorly and adducts on the right femoral head. Simultaneously, the right innominate anteriorly rotates and the left innominate posteriorly rotates driving the sacrum into left rotation. The sacrum counternutates at the right sacroiliac joint and nutates at the left. The hamstring muscles relax and the gluteus maximus muscle becomes more active (Inman et al 1981). This occurs in conjunction with a counter rotation of the trunk and firing of the contralateral latissimus dorsi muscle (Gracovetsky 1997, Vleeming et al 1997). Together, these two muscles tense the thoracodorsal fascia and facilitate the force

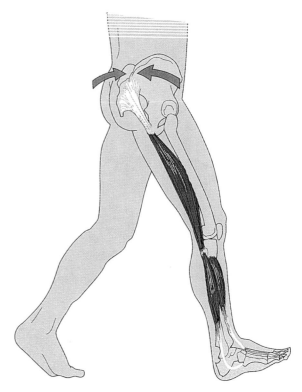

Figure 5.39 At heel strike, posterior rotation of the right innominate increases the tension of the right sacrotuberous ligament. Contraction of the biceps femoris further increases tension in this ligament preparing the sacroiliac joint for impact. (Redrawn from Vleeming et al 1997.)

closure mechanism through the sacroiliac joint (Fig. 5.40). The superincumbent body weight is thereby transferred to the lower extremity through a system which is stabilized through ligamentous and myofascial tension.

From heel strike through midstance, the ipsilateral gluteus medius and the contralateral adductors are active to stabilize the pelvic girdle on the femoral heads. Muscle activity is much less in all groups during the double support phase since both legs receive the body weight. In optimal gait, the center of gravity travels along a smooth sinusoidal curve both vertically and laterally. The displacement in both planes should be no more than 5 cm (Inman et al 1981).

The displacement of the center of gravity is exaggerated when the pelvic girdle is unable to transfer load (insufficient in either form closure or force closure) (Lee 1997a). The patient

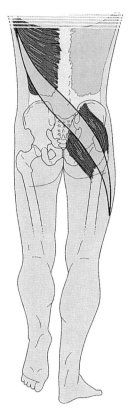

Figure 5.40 During the right single-leg stance phase, contraction of the gluteus maximus and the contralateral latissimus dorsi increases tension through the thoracodorsal fascia and facilitates continued stability of the sacroiliac joint during the weight-bearing phase.

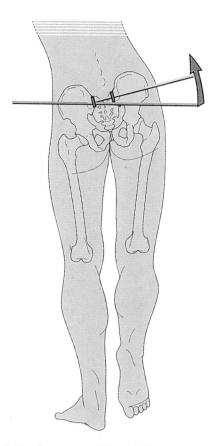

Figure 5.41 Compensated Trendelenburg.

attempts to compensate by reducing the forces through the pelvic girdle. In a fully compensated gait, the patient transfers their weight laterally over the involved limb (compensated Trendelenburg) thus reducing the vertical shear forces through the sacroiliac joint (Fig. 5.41). In a non-compensated gait pattern, the patient tends to demonstrate a true Trendelenburg (Fig. 5.42). The pelvic girdle adducts excessively (on the weight-bearing leg). The femur abducts relative to the foot thus bringing the center of gravity closer to the sacroiliac joint which reduces the vertical shear force.

Lumbar vertebrae

During gait, the lower lumbar vertebrae rotate in the same sense as the sacrum. This axis about which lumbar rotation occurs is oblique (see Fig. 5.5) such that contralateral sideflexion and forward flexion occur in conjunction with the rotation (Bogduk 1997, Gracovetsky & Farfan 1986). The iliolumbar ligament modifies this motion at the L5–S1 segment (Fig. 5.6) (Pearcy & Tibrewal 1984). In most individuals, the total available range of motion at the lumbosacral junction is not utilized in walking and minor restrictions may not be apparent objectively, nor felt subjectively, during prolonged walking.

In conclusion, patients presenting with a primary lumbosacral joint dysfunction rarely complain of difficulty in walking whereas those presenting with pelvic girdle and/or hip disorders often state that walking is their most aggravating activity. It is recognized that the study of gait is incomplete without considering

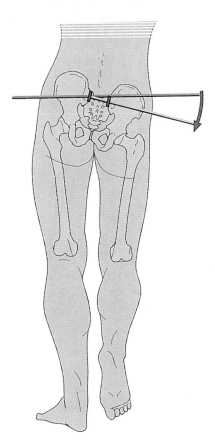

Figure 5.42 True Trendelenburg.

the influences of the foot and knee on both habitual and compensatory gait patterns at the lumbo-pelvic-hip region; however, this subject shall be left for the reader to explore once the basics are understood.

6

Pain and dysfunction/the healing process

PAIN AND DYSFUNCTION

In the late 1970s and early 1980s, the emphasis of manual therapy was on the detection and treatment of painful joints. Using specific manual techniques it was possible to identify the painful cervical zygapophyseal joints 100% of the time in a blind study with diagnostic anaesthetic joint blocks (Jull et al 1988). It is apparent from this study that the technique tested was valid and specific.

Formal studies using intra-articular anaesthetic joint blocks have shown a prevalence of pain coming from the sacroiliac joint in 15–21% of people with low back pain (Maigne et al 1996, Schwarzer et al 1995). Recently (Maigne et al 1996), an attempt was made to assess the validity of certain manual techniques which were thought to provoke pain from the sacroiliac joint. Of 67 participants, 54 had at least 75% of their pain relieved when the sacroiliac joint was injected under fluoroscopy. All participants had suffered from their pain for more than 50 days. These subjects then had several sacroiliac pain provocation tests applied to their pelvic girdle; the response was noted and correlated with the findings from the joint block. The tests investigated included distraction, compression, sacral pressure, Gaenslen, Patrick, pain on resisted external rotation of the hip and pressure directly over the pubic symphysis. The result reported was that: 'There was no statistically significant association between response to blocks and any single clinical parameter. No pain provocation test was a useful predictor of sacroiliac joint pain' (Maigne et al 1996).

Dreyfuss et al (1996) were also unsuccessful in identifying either a consistent medical history or relevant sacroiliac joint test (as determined by a multidisciplinary expert panel) which was useful in detecting those people who had 90% of their pain relieved with anaesthetic joint blocks. The tests in this study included:

1. pain drawing depicting pain over the sacroiliac joint
2. pain drawing depicting pain into the buttock
3. pain drawing depicting pain into the groin
4. pointing to within 2 measured inches of the PSIS to indicate the site of maximal pain
5. sitting with partial elevation from the chair of the buttock on the affected side
6. Gillet test
7. thigh thrust
8. Patrick's test
9. Gaenslen's test
10. midline sacral thrust
11. sacral sulcus tenderness
12. joint play.

They emphatically state that 'The results of the present study vindicate [these] reservations and offer little support to proponents of the use of physical examination for diagnosis.' This belief is supported internationally by respected authors in this subject (Bogduk 1997, Buyruk et al 1997, Laslett 1997, Mooney 1997, Vleeming et al 1997). Bogduk's (1997) interpretation of this work is that 'although sacroiliac joint pain is common in patients with chronic low back pain, it can only be diagnosed using diagnostic local anaesthetic blocks.'

Perhaps we have not yet 'discovered' the right manual tests for the sacroiliac joint. How can we be so accurate with respect to the cervical spine and so inaccurate in the pelvic girdle? Dreyfuss et al (1996) put forth this challenge: 'If proponents of other tests believe that their tests are superior, they have the responsibility and the means to validate those tests by challenging them with diagnostic, intra-articular sacroiliac joint blocks as described in this study.' There are

better tests (Lee 1992) which are more specific to the sacroiliac joint but they evaluate function, not pain, and this is where the paradigm has gone wrong. Pain does not equal dysfunction.

Pain is an emotional experience which depends on many biopsychosocial factors. Those which initiate the pain response (mechanical and/or chemical deformation of nociceptors in pain-sensitive tissues) can be quite different from those which maintain the perception. Pain disability is a form of pain behavior (Vlaeyen et al 1997) constantly influenced by environmental conditions. According to Vlaeyen et al (1997) pain disability shifts from a structural/mechanical control to a cognitive/environmental control over a period of 4–8 weeks. All of the subjects in the two studies noted above had their pain for longer than 8 weeks.

The word 'dys' is Greek for abnormal, the word 'function' is Latin for performance. Abnormal performance has nothing to do with pain perception. Many people have abnormal joint function (stiffness-arthrodesis, looseness-instability) and no pain from these joints. Others have apparently full function in terms of mobility and stability and yet intra-articular joint blocks relieve their pain (Buyruk et al 1997). Stiff joints put extra stress on those above and below them, and over time symptoms may appear. Maigne et al (1996) do concede that 'It remains possible that a major part of the so-called sacroiliac pathology is a pathology of the soft tissues surrounding the joint.' Or maybe, the joints above and/or below the ones which are *dysfunctional* are responsible for the pain.

In the early 1980s the osteopathic approach to musculoskeletal medicine was introduced to physiotherapists in Canada. The biomechanical model was received with enthusiasm and quickly replaced therapy based on pain models. The first edition of this text presented a biomechanical approach to the assessment and treatment of dysfunction (not pain) of the lumbo-pelvic-hip region which reflected the knowledge available at the time. While the model of function has improved, validation of functional tests has been lacking (Carmichael 1987, Dreyfuss et al 1994, 1996, Herzog et al 1989,

Laslett 1994, Paydar et al 1994, Potter & Rothstein 1985). Physical examination of the knee joint is a well accepted form of diagnosis of mechanical dysfunction. There is no reason why physical examination of the sacroiliac joint cannot evolve once better tests are developed.

When treating *dysfunction*, it is important to restore the optimal biomechanics so that the injured soft tissue which may be responsible for nociception can heal (White & Sahrmann 1994).

THE HEALING PROCESS

When an injury has occurred either directly (macrotrauma over a short period of time) or indirectly (microtrauma over a long period of time) to the soft tissues of the body, the principles of treatment follow those of the body's natural healing process. Since it is doubtful that anything can be done to accelerate the normal response, the intent of therapy is to prevent and/or reverse the factors which tend to retard recovery. The aim is to restore the biomechanics and then treat the soft tissue according to the stage of its recovery.

Approximately three billion years ago when living organisms were unicellular, death of the cell meant death of the organism. With the evolution of multicellular organisms, so followed the process of repair after injury. Ultimately this repair process was perfected so that complete regeneration of an amputated limb was possible. Some lower vertebrates such as lizards and newts have retained this capability. The evolution of more complex life forms (e.g. the mammal) has occurred at the expense of total regenerative ability. For example, in man, cardiac muscle does not regenerate after infarction, neural tissue does not regenerate after cellular death, skin does not regenerate after full-thickness injury and an amputated finger does not grow back. With few exceptions mammalian tissue responds to injury by repair rather than regeneration.

In most tissues, repair occurs by fibrous tissue proliferation regardless of which tissue has been damaged. Although the healing process is not a state it can be divided into three phases—the substrate phase, the fibroblastic phase and maturation.

Substrate phase

The substrate phase (also called the lag, latent or productive phase) extends from the time of injury to the 4th to 6th day. It is characterized by the inflammatory response which prepares the wound for subsequent healing by removing the debris, necrotic tissue and bacteria. At the same time, fibroblasts migrate to the wound site. Exactly how these cells are attracted to the wound is unknown; however, several investigators (Bassett 1968, Kappel et al 1973, Peacock 1984) feel that an electric potential exists at the injury site which influences their migration. During this phase, the wound is held together by the gluing action of fibrin which has a very low breaking strength.

Fibroblastic phase

The fibroblastic phase begins between the 4th and 6th day after injury and can last up to 4 to 10 weeks (Peacock 1984). At this time, the proliferating fibroblasts begin to synthesize collagen, mucopolysaccharides and glyco-proteins. Regardless of the location of the wound, the fibroblasts carry on the process of wound repair by replacing the damaged structures with fibrous tissue. Tropocollagen is secreted from the fibroblasts and quickly aggregates into collagen fibers. The orientation of the fibers at this stage has been shown (Bassett 1968, Peacock 1984) to be influenced by the mechanical forces existing at the wound site. The tensile strength of the wound during the fibroblastic phase is proportional to the quantity of collagen present rather than the cross-linking between the collagen fibers.

Maturation phase

These is no sharp demarcation between the end of the fibroblastic phase and the beginning of the maturation phase. Peacock (1984) states that the quantity of collagen within the wound ceases to increase between the 3rd and 4th week after injury. Although the collagen content within the wound remains constant or even decreases after the stage of fibroplasia, the wound continues to gain in tensile strength. This strength gain is due to two factors: the intra-molecular/inter-molecular cross-linking of the collagen fibers, and remodeling of the wound by the dissolution and reformation of the collagen fibers to give a stronger weave. The quantity of collagen is constant; it is the organization that is undergoing change. This process of remodeling may require 6 to 12 months for completion.

Clinical application to treatment

Much of the functional disability seen within the musculoskeletal system is caused by the synthesis and deposition of scar tissue and the way in which the physical properties of collagen differ from the unwounded tissue it replaces. The therapist must therefore be aware of the ultimate function of the injured tissue, otherwise no assessment can be made of the efficacy of repair or the long-term effect. In other words, repair, while restoring structure, may seriously interfere with function. For example, the fibrous tissue which replaces ruptured muscle fibers is non-contractile, less extensible and cannot replace the function of the torn myofiber. The aim of treatment therefore, must be to control and to guide the repair process such that optimal structure and function are restored. Unfortunately, this is not always possible.

Can anything be done to accelerate the normal rate of healing? During the stage of fibroplasia, the tensile strength of the wound is proportional to the rate of collagen accumulation. Webster et al (1980) have shown that ultrasound can increase the quantity of collagen synthesized, thereby increasing the tensile strength of the scar. Research (Abergel 1984, Mester 1971) on the effects of lasers indicates that facilitation of the optimal rate of healing is possible with this modality. However, whether it is possible to shorten the total length of time required for maturation of the scar is controversial. What can be done, however, is to prevent the undesirable

factors which tend to retard the healing process. The fibrosis can also be controlled and directed during the stages of synthesis, deposition and remodeling, such that a more functional scar subserves the tissue it replaces as best it can.

Tendon

To illustrate, compare the structural characteristics of the tendon of the piriformis muscle with those of the peroneus longus muscle. The tendon of piriformis is relatively short and is not enclosed in a synovial sheath (Fig. 6.1). The collagen fibers within the tendon are oriented in a longitudinal regular manner (Fig. 6.2), consistent with the lines of stress produced when the muscle contracts. Since the Type I collagen which is present in tendon is inelastic, this arrangement allows the force generated by contraction of the muscle to be efficiently transmitted to the bony insertion on the greater trochanter. Minimal gliding of the tendon on the adjacent structures is required for normal function.

Conversely, the tendon of the peroneus longus muscle is long and is enclosed within a synovial sheath passing beneath several fibrous tunnels on the lateral aspect of the ankle as well as

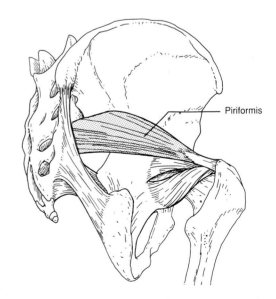

Figure 6.1 The piriformis muscle and its tendon.

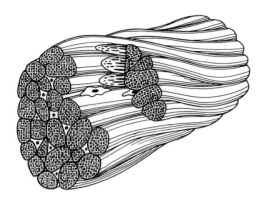

Figure 6.2 Both tendons and ligaments are composed of a regular longitudinal arrangement of collagen fibers. (Redrawn from Warwick & Williams 1989.)

within the sole of the foot (Fig. 6.3). The collagen fibers within the tendon are also oriented in a longitudinal manner (Fig. 6.2) consistent with the lines of stress produced when the muscle contracts. Again, this arrangement facilitates the transmission of force from the muscle belly to the bone efficiently. However, when the muscle contracts, the tendon is required to glide extensively between the adjacent structures and the restoration of this function is critical to the success of treatment.

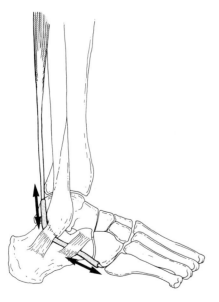

Figure 6.3 The peroneus longus muscle, its tendon and synovial sheath.

The repair process following injury to either of these tendons is the same. The inflammatory response of the substrate phase is followed by the proliferation of fibroblasts and the production of collagen, mucopolysaccharides and glycoproteins. The orientation of the new collagen fibers at this stage of repair is influenced by mechanical deformation of the wound. Exactly how tension effects the orientation process is controversial; however, research (Bassett 1968, Kappel et al 1973) suggests that the electrical field surrounding the injury site may influence both healing and regeneration of tissue.

In 1880, Pierre and Jacques Curie discovered that when a quartz crystal was stressed, a potential difference was produced across its faces. This was called the piezoelectric effect. It is felt (Bassett 1968, Kappel et al 1973, Peacock 1984) that since collagen is crystalline in nature, a potential difference, or field of electricity, is produced when the fibers are deformed. Perhaps this deformation produces the piezoelectric current which subsequently directs the newly formed collagen fibrils. Bassett (1968) has described the cellular effects of electrical current and believes these to be the trigger of wound repair. Clinically, this appears to be the most effective stage in which to implement electrical, ultrasonic, light and/or manual therapy if optimal function is to be achieved.

The tendons of the piriformis and peroneus longus muscles contain Type 1 collagen fibers which lie in a longitudinal direction in series with the muscle fibers. Therefore, during the fibroblastic stage of healing, treatment should be directed towards orienting the collagen fibres of both tendons longitudinally. Passive physiological mobilizations and exercise programs which *gently* stress the tendon should be started at this stage. Vigorous exercises or aggressive passive mobilizations will prevent the revascularization of the tendon and retard the healing process, so 'gentle' is the key word at this time. As well, since there is minimal intra-molecular or inter-molecular cross-linking of collagen fibers at this stage, strong stretching or forcing of the wound is contraindicated. More pain will definitely lead to less gain. Both ultrasound and laser can facilitate the synthesis of collagen and are useful adjunctive modalities.

The maturation phase is the stage when things can definitely go wrong. The structure may be restored and extremely resistant to tensile forces but the function may be completely devastated. Consider the torn peroneus longus tendon in the foot. Collagen cannot differentiate between the tendon, the synovium and the fibrous tunnel. The new collagen fibers uniting the tendon will indiscriminately cross-link with those restoring the structure of the sheath or the fibrous tunnel beneath which it passes. Stability is thus restored at the expense of mobility. Since this tendon must glide extensively for normal function, a 50% reduction in the gliding ability will have profound effects on the function of the foot. By contrast, the tendon of the piriformis muscle requires little mobility between itself and the adjacent structures, and loss of this mobility will have less effect on the overall function.

There are two kinds of adhesions which can occur subsequent to the healing process, restrictive and non-restrictive. Restrictive adhesions are regularly organized with a compact arrangement of collagen fibers oriented in a longitudinal manner. Non-restrictive adhesions are randomly organized with small fiber bundles. Although the evidence is not conclusive, it is felt (Peacock 1984) that longitudinal slippage or friction-induced instability of collagen fibers and fibrils is the most probable method by which additional length in the scar is gained.

This information can be applied to healing tissue in the following manner. If the injured tendon is stressed repetitively during the therapeutic exercise program, an excellent environment will be created for lateral inter-tissue cross-linking. This facilitates tensile strength but a restrictive adhesion will also be encouraged. If, however, transverse mobilizations (or frictions) of the tendon are also incorporated into the therapy session, elongation of the entire adhesion will be promoted as the collagen fibers are 'teased' apart and longitudinal slippage of the fibers occurs. The adhesion is therefore non-

restrictive and both tensile strength and mobility are encouraged.

To summarize, tendon tensile strength can be effectively restored by exercise programs which apply stress to the tendon. These programs can be graduated from gentle passive stretching to vigorous eccentric loading depending upon the stage of healing. If tendon mobility is also required, attention must be directed to the lateral attachments which bind the tendon down, otherwise the stage is set for chronic repeated microtears of scar tissue such as those seen in chronic tennis elbow or chronic peroneal tendinitis following old inversion injuries of the ankle.

Ligament

Ligaments structurally resemble tendons and therefore the tensile requirements are the same. They must, however, be free to move on the bones they cross. If a restrictive adhesion is allowed to develop, chronic repeated microtears will occur. If the adhesion can be elongated via transverse frictions, the mobility and the elasticity of the ligament will be restored. Manipulation of adhesions is a destructive treatment technique since the adhesion rarely releases where it is intended. More commonly, a fresh tear between the adhesion and normal tissue occurs which sets up another inflammatory response. If the fibroblastic phase and the maturation phase of collagen synthesis, deposition and remodeling are now treated appropriately, a new elongated adhesion will be formed which allows the necessary mobility.

Fibrous joint capsule

The structural characteristics and functional requirements of a fibrous joint capsule are quite different from those of either a tendon or ligament. The outer layer of the joint capsule is composed of an irregular random arrangement of collagen fibers (Fig. 6.4) unlike the tendon or ligament which displays a regular longitudinal arrangement (Fig. 6.2). This is a good example of function governing structure. The primary

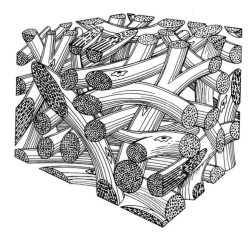

Figure 6.4 The outer layer of the joint capsule is composed of an irregular random arrangement of collagen fibers. (Redrawn from Warwick & Williams 1989.)

function of a ligament is to resist tensile forces between two bones, and the anatomy suits its needs ideally. The fibrous capsule, however, must be extensible to allow mobility of the joint, and since collagen is inextensible a longitudinal arrangement would inhibit mobility.

The random, irregular orientation of the collagen fibers permits mobility. When the capsule is stretched, the fibers orient themselves along the lines of tension produced by the stretch. Ultimately, the collagen fibers set the limit to the amount of extensibility permitted (Fig. 6.5). This anatomical arrangement promotes mobility

while the physical characteristics of the collagen fiber itself afford end-range stability.

The repair process following capsular injury is identical to the one previously described. The initial inflammatory response is clinically apparent as traumatic arthritis. Fibroplasia and collagen synthesis follows 4 to 6 days after injury. The orientation of the new fibers will not automatically assume a random arrangement if tensile forces are applied to the wound. If the patient is started on an exercise program designed to restore full range of motion, and that exercise program puts tension through the wound, longitudinal orientation of new collagen fibers will be promoted leading to increased lateral cross-linking and restricted mobility. This is not an adhesion, but rather the restoration of structure with tissue that does not subserve the joint capsule's function. The treatment given to any tissue is governed by the functional requirements of the damaged tissue. In this instance, both extensibility and tensile strength require restoration.

The challenge is to preserve the extensibility of the joint capsule by creating a random arrangement of small-fiber collagen bundles while simultaneously increasing the tensile strength. An extensible scar is more likely to develop if stresses are induced in a multitude of directions across the wound. Three-dimensional exercise programs, together with physiological

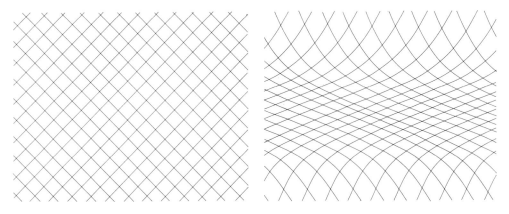

Figure 6.5 The orientation of the collagen fibers within the joint capsule influences the degree of extensibility permitted. The random irregular orientation initially permits mobility (left). When placed under tension the reorientation of the fibers (right) ultimately restricts the motion.

active and passive mobilization techniques, will theoretically facilitate the random arrangement of the new collagen fibers. Unidirectional passive accessory joint mobilizations applied for 30 seconds to 3 minutes would be counter-productive since they would stress the wound longitudinally and subsequently facilitate a longitudinal arrangement of the collagen fibers. This would actually restrict the joint mobility. It is difficult to believe, however, that even 15 minutes of passive articular mobilization could have a lasting influence on the ultimate orientation of collagen within the scar tissue since healing is a 24-hour process. Thus there is need for appropriate exercise programs and patient involvement in their own rehabilitation.

SUMMARY

Left alone, wounded tissue will repair. The efficacy of the repair process depends on how well the replacement tissue restores the tissue's original function and what effect this restoration has on the biomechanics of the region. The resolution of the pain which accompanies the injury depends on many biopsychosocial factors. If during the injury process the biomechanics of the lumbo-pelvic-hip region have been altered, the patient may compensate for dysfunction in many ways. The onset of decompensation pain may occur several days, months or years later. The role of therapy is not to treat pain but to restore the biomechanics and then guide the deposition and remodeling of any healing tissue at each stage of repair. To achieve this, it is paramount that the patients become active participants in their rehabilitation programs.

7

Subjective and objective examination

Dysfunction of the lumbo-pelvic-hip region implies abnormal performance, according to the classical derivations of the words 'dys' and 'function'. When a biomechanical model is used to treat patients with dysfunction, the location and behavior of pain becomes less relevant to the assessment and subsequent treatment planning. However, to ignore completely the patient's complaints is to fail to address the psychosocial factors of pain. Dreyfuss et al (1996) note 'Patients with sacroiliac joint pain exhibit no characteristic feature such as aggravation or relief of their pain by sitting, walking, standing, flexion, or extension.' This finding is not surprising if pain is used to indicate dysfunction (see Ch. 6). Clinically, events which tend to aggravate and relieve symptoms follow common patterns when patients with similar dysfunctions (not pain) are considered. Thus, it is important to investigate the symptom behavior as this will address the patient's psychosocial needs as well as provide a preliminary indication of the underlying dysfunction once clinical expertise is attained. Therapists who take the time to develop a disciplined examination technique will be rewarded later with the ability to recognize similar patterns of dysfunction quickly. The purpose of this section is to describe and illustrate the basic subjective and objective examination which should be part of every assessment.

SUBJECTIVE EXAMINATION (Table 7.1)

Mode of onset

- How did the problem begin: suddenly or insidiously? With respect to wound repair, is the patient presenting during the substrate, fibroblastic or maturation phase of healing?
- Was there an element of trauma? If so, was there a major traumatic event over a short period of time, such as a fall, or was there a series of minor traumatic events over a prolonged period of time, such as the habitual use of improper lifting technique?
- Is this the first episode requiring treatment or has there been a similar past history of events? If this is a repeat episode, how long did it take to recover from the previous one and was therapy necessary at that time?

Pain/dysaesthesia

- Exactly where is the pain/dysaesthesia? Is it localized or diffuse and can its quality be described?
- How far down the limb or limbs do the symptoms radiate?
- Which activities (including how much) will aggravate the symptoms?
- What effect do prolonged sitting, standing, walking, stair-climbing and descent, rolling over in bed, getting in/out of a chair/car,

cough and/or sneeze have on the pain/dysaesthesia?
- Which activities (including how much) provide relief?

Sleep

- Are the symptoms interfering with sleep? Does rest provide relief?
- What kind of bed is being slept in and what position is most frequently adopted?

Occupation/leisure activities/sport

- What level of physical activity does the patient consider as normal and essential for return to full function?
- What are the patient's goals from therapy? The specifics of both the patient's occupation and sport are required if rehabilitation is to be successful and complete.

General information

- What is the status of the patient's general health?
- Is the patient currently taking any medication for this or any other condition?
- What are the results of any adjunctive diagnostic tests (i.e. X-ray, computerized tomography (CT) scan, magnetic resonance imaging (MRI), laboratory tests, etc.)?

Table 7.1 Subjective examination

NAME	AGE	DR
MODE OF ONSET		
PAST HISTORY	PAST TREATMENT	
PAIN/DYSAESTHESIA Location	Aggravating activities Relief activities	
SLEEP Surface/position	Status in a.m.	
OCCUPATION/LEISURE ACTIVITIES/SPORT		
GENERAL HEALTH	MEDICATION	
RESULTS OF ADJUNCTIVE TESTS		

OBJECTIVE EXAMINATION (Table 7.2)

The objective examination includes gait and postural analysis, evaluation of functional tests, specific tests of articular mobility and stability, muscle function, neurological, vascular and adjunctive tests.

Bogduk (1997) states that biomechanical diagnoses require biomechanical criteria. He notes that 'Pain on movement is not that criteria.' Tests which aim to analyse the mobility and stability of a joint are required to fulfill these criteria. Recently, several biomechanical tests of the sacroiliac joint have been criticized with regard to their reliability, validity and specificity (Bogduk 1997, Buyruk et al 1997, Carmichael 1987, Dreyfuss et al 1994, 1996, Herzog et al 1989, Laslett 1994, 1997, Maigne et al 1996, Paydar et al 1994, Potter & Rothstein 1985). From this research, it has been suggested that manual testing of the sacroiliac joint is unreliable and therefore should be abandoned. This conclusion has not been reached with other joints of the body. Stability tests for the knee joint (Lachman's and the anterior drawer tests) are commonly accepted amongst both physiotherapists and orthopaedic surgeons (Reid 1992) even though their reliability, validity and specificity have been questioned (Cooperman et al 1990). The results from the latter inter-tester reliability study clearly showed poor agreement in all areas. In spite of this research, the Lachman's test remains widely used for evaluation of stability at the knee joint. Biomechanical diagnoses require biomechanical criteria; the presence of pain on movement is not one (Bogduk 1997).

The tests for spinal and sacroiliac joint function (i.e. mobility/stability, not pain) continue to be developed and hopefully will be able to withstand the scrutiny and rigor of scientific research and take their place in a clinical evaluation which follows a biomechanical and not a pain model. The tests are presented with good intention, recognizing their failure to respond in isolation to reliability and validity studies. They remain the best we have and when a clinical reasoning process is applied to their findings, a logical biomechanical diagnosis can

Table 7.2 Objective examination

GAIT	POSTURE

FUNCTIONAL TESTS
Standing: forward/backward bending
    Lumbosacral junction
    Pelvic girdle
Standing: squat
Standing: lateral bending
Standing: striding
    Ipsilateral posterior rotation test (Gillet)
    Ipsilateral anterior rotation test
Sitting: functional hamstring length
Sitting: functional thoracodorsal fascial length
Supine: active straight leg raise
Prone: active straight leg raise

ARTICULAR MOBILITY/STABILITY TESTS
Lumbosacral junction: positional tests
Lumbosacral junction: osteokinematic tests of physiological mobility
    Flexion/extension
    Sideflexion/rotation
Lumbosacral junction: arthrokinematic tests of accessory joint mobility
    Superoanterior glide
    Inferoposterior glide
Lumbosacral junction: arthrokinetic tests of stability/stress
    Compression
    Torsion
    Posteroanterior shear
    Anteroposterior shear
Pelvic girdle: positional tests
    Innominate
    Sacrum
Pelvic girdle: arthrokinematic tests of accessory joint mobility
    Inferoposterior glide innominate/sacrum
    Superoanterior glide innominate/sacrum
Pelvic girdle: arthrokinetic tests of stability
    Anteroposterior translation: innominate/sacrum
    Superoinferior translation: innominate/sacrum
    Superoinferior: pubic symphysis
Pain provocation tests
    Transverse anterior distraction: posterior compression
    Transverse posterior distraction: anterior compression
    Long dorsal sacroiliac ligament
    Sacrotuberous/interosseous ligaments
Hip: osteokinematic tests of physiological mobility
    Flexion
    Extension
    Abduction
    Adduction
    Lateral rotation
    Medial rotation
    Quadrant test
Hip: arthrokinematic tests of accessory joint mobility
    Lateral/medial translation
    Distraction/compression
    Anteroposterior/posteroanterior glide

Cont'd overpage

Table 7.2   *Cont'd*

GAIT	POSTURE
Hip: arthrokinetic tests of stability	
Proprioception	
Torque test	
Iliofemoral ligament	
Pubofemoral ligament	
Ischiofemoral ligament	

MUSCLE FUNCTION TESTS

Muscle recruitment/strength: inner unit
   Transversus abdominis
   Multifidus
   Levator ani
Muscle recruitment/strength: outer unit
   Posterior oblique system
   Anterior oblique system
   Lateral system
Muscle length
   Erector spinae
   Hamstrings
   Rectus femoris
   Iliopsoas
   Tensor fascia lata
   Adductors
   Piriformis
Contractile lesions

NEUROLOGICAL TESTS

Motor   Sensory   Reflex
Dural mobility

VASCULAR TESTS

ADJUNCTIVE TEST RESULTS

SUMMARY

be made. Without apology, they continue to be defended.

Gait

Careful observation of the patient's gait can be informative since walking requires optimal lumbo-pelvic-hip function (see Ch. 5). In particular, deviation of the center of gravity in the vertical and/or transverse planes or alteration in stride length and timing can be indicative of kinematic and/or kinetic dysfunction within the lumbo-pelvic-hip complex.

Posture

Postural asymmetry is not necessarily indicative of pelvic girdle dysfunction; however, pelvic girdle dysfunction is often reflected via postural asymmetry. Therefore, postural analysis in relation to the sagittal, coronal and transverse planes of the body is essential. In particular, careful observation of the distribution of body weight through the lower quadrant is required.

Ideally, if the body is viewed from the lateral aspect, a vertical line should pass through the following points (Fig. 7.1):

1. the external auditory meatus
2. the bodies of the cervical vertebrae
3. the glenohumeral joint
4. slightly anterior to the bodies of the thoracic vertebrae, transecting the vertebrae at the thoracolumbar junction
5. the bodies of the lumbar vertebrae
6. the sacral promontory
7. slightly posterior to the coronal axis of the hip joint

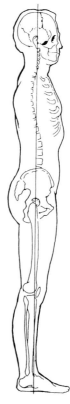

Figure 7.1   Position of optimal postural balance in standing. (Reproduced with permission from Lee & Walsh 1996.)

8. slightly anterior to the coronal axis of the knee joint
9. slightly anterior to the talocrural joint
10. the naviculo calcaneo-cuboid joint.

Functional tests

These tests examine the integrated motor control of the lower quadrant and specifically the ability to transfer load. They require optimal function of the active (force closure) and passive (form closure) systems according to Panjabi's model (1992) (Fig. 5.13). The tests chosen reflect the clinical application of the biomechanical model presented in Chapter 5. A diagnosis cannot be made on the findings of one test alone. A clinical reasoning process which incorporates the findings of all of the tests is necessary to reach a mechanical diagnosis. These tests lead the examiner to further evaluation of the active and passive systems when dysfunction is noted.

Standing: forward and backward bending

Lumbosacral junction (flexion/extension) (Fig. 7.2). With the patient standing with his/her weight equally distributed through both lower limbs, the L5 segment is palpated bilaterally. The patient is instructed to forward/backward bend

and the symmetry of motion of the transverse processes is noted. Neither rotation nor sideflexion of the L5 vertebra should occur coupled with flexion/extension during forward or backward bending (see Fig. 5.2).

Pelvic girdle (Lee & Walsh 1996). This is a useful preliminary test of pelvic girdle function since asymmetry of motion is present in *all* unilateral hypomobile disorders of the sacroiliac and/or hip joint. However, asymmetry of motion during this test does not mean that the sacroiliac joint is hypomobile. A finding can be reported but a judgement cannot be made from one test alone.

Asymmetric intra-pelvic motion is detected in the following manner (Fig. 7.3). With the patient standing with his/her weight equally distributed through both lower limbs, the inferior aspect of the posterior superior iliac spine (PSIS) is palpated bilaterally. The patient is instructed to forward bend and the symmetry of motion of the PSISs is noted. The PSISs should move equally in a superior direction. The patient is then instructed to backward bend and the symmetry of motion of the PSISs is noted. They should move equally in an inferior direction.

The relative flexibility of the longitudinal system and the timing of sacral nutation/counternutation during forward bending of the trunk is tested as follows. With the patient standing with his/her weight equally

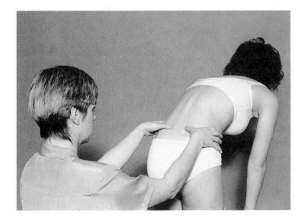

Figure 7.2 Active physiological mobility test for flexion/extension of the lumbosacral junction. The transverse processes of the L5 vertebra should travel an equal distance in a superior direction.

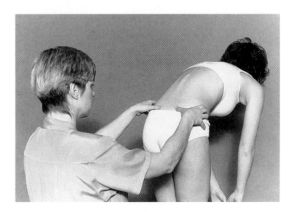

Figure 7.3 Active physiological mobility test for forward bending of the innominates. The PSISs should travel an equal distance in a superior direction.

distributed through both lower limbs, the inferior aspect of the PSIS is palpated with one thumb while the other palpates the sacral base directly parallel (Fig. 7.4). The patient is instructed to forward bend. The sacral base commonly moves anterior relative to the PSIS during the first 45° of forward bending (sacral nutation). At some point after this, the sacrum will stop moving and the innominate will rotate anteriorly relative to the sacrum (sacral counternutation). The further in the range this occurs, the more stable the sacroiliac joint. For the sacrum to nutate bilaterally, it must be able to glide inferoposteriorly relative to the innominate at both sacroiliac joints (Fig. 5.8). The sacrum should remain in a nutated position relative to

the innominates during backward bending of the trunk.

Standing: squat

The ability of the hip joint to obtain and to bear full weight in flexion is tested by asking the patient to perform a bilateral and/or unilateral squat.

Standing: lateral bending

With the patient standing with his/her weight equally distributed through both lower limbs, he/she is instructed to laterally bend to alternate sides (see Fig. 5.33). The ability of the pelvic girdle to translate laterally to the opposite side without deviation is noted.

Standing: striding (intra-pelvic torsion)

This test is also known as the Gillet test and examines the ability of the pelvis to twist (see Fig. 5.32) as well as the ability to transfer weight through the pelvic girdle during unipedal stance.

Ipsilateral posterior rotation test (Gillet) (Fig. 7.5) (Lee & Walsh 1996). With the patient standing with his/her weight evenly distributed through both lower limbs, the inferior aspect of the PSIS is palpated with one thumb while the other palpates the sacral base directly parallel. The patient is instructed to flex the ipsilateral femur at the hip joint and the inferomedial displacement of the PSIS relative to the sacrum is noted.

Attention should also be directed to the patient's ability to transfer weight through the contralateral limb and to maintain balance. Kinetic dysfunction is often revealed at this point. The test is then repeated on and compared with the opposite side.

The right ipsilateral posterior rotation test examines the ability of the right innominate to posteriorly rotate, the sacrum to right rotate and the L5 vertebra to right rotate/sideflex (see Fig. 5.32). The innominate must be free to glide anterosuperiorly relative to the sacrum at the right sacroiliac joint (Fig. 5.11).

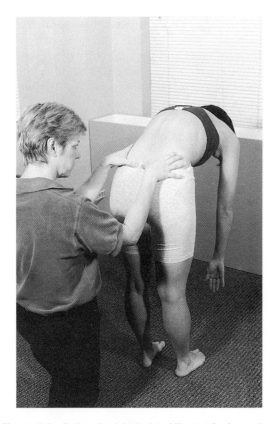

Figure 7.4 Active physiological mobility test for forward bending of the sacrum. The sacrum should remain in nutation throughout this test. In some, a slight increase in motion can be felt at the beginning of the range followed by a relative counternutation at the end. In this case, the timing of sacral counternutation is noted.

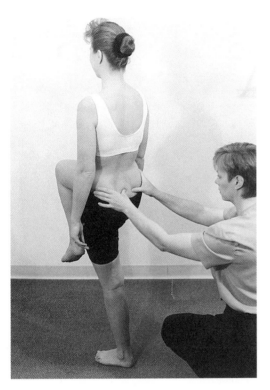

Figure 7.5 Ipsilateral posterior rotation test (Gillet). Note the inferomedial displacement of the PSIS.

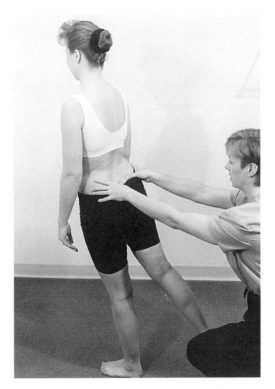

Figure 7.6 Ipsilateral anterior rotation test. Note the superolateral displacement of the PSIS.

Ipsilateral anterior rotation test (Fig. 7.6) (Lee & Walsh 1996). With the patient standing with his/her weight evenly distributed through both lower limbs, the inferior aspect of the PSIS is palpated with one thumb while the other palpates the sacral base directly parallel. The patient is instructed to extend the ipsilateral femur at the hip joint and the superolateral displacement of the PSIS relative to the sacrum is noted.

The right ipsilateral anterior rotation test examines the ability of the right innominate to anteriorly rotate, the sacrum to left rotate and the L5 vertebra to left rotate/sideflex. The innominate must be free to glide inferoposteriorly relative to the sacrum at the right sacroiliac joint (Fig. 5.10).

Sitting: functional hamstring length (Fig. 7.7)

With the patient sitting in a neutral lumbar spine position, the inferior aspect of the PSIS is palpated with one thumb while the other palpates the sacral base directly parallel. The patient is instructed to extend the knee and the ability to do so without posteriorly rotating the pelvic girdle or flexing the lumbar spine is noted. An extensible hamstring should allow full extension of the knee without any motion occurring in the lumbar spine or pelvic girdle.

Sitting: functional thoracodorsal fascia length (Fig. 7.8)

The patient sits in a neutral lumbar spine position with their arms resting by their sides. They are instructed to rotate the trunk to the left and then to the right and the quantity and quality of motion through the lumbar spine and pelvic girdle is noted. Subsequently, they are instructed to flex their arms to 90° and fully externally rotate and adduct their shoulders such that the hypothenar eminences are

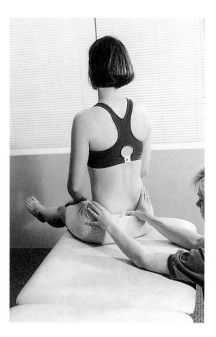

Figure 7.7 Test of functional length of the deep longitudinal system (hamstrings and the sacrotuberous ligament).

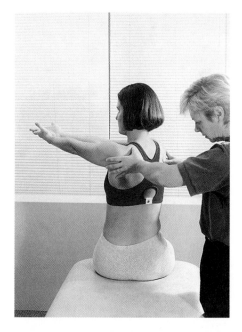

Figure 7.8 Test of functional length of the thoracodorsal fascia and the latissimus dorsi muscle. The range of motion of trunk rotation is compared with and without the system under stretch.

approximated. This position increases the tension through the latissimus dorsi muscle (Kendall et al 1993). From this position, they are instructed to rotate the trunk to the left and then to the right. The quantity and quality of the motion is noted and compared to that observed with the arms by the side. The motion is markedly reduced in this position when the thoracodorsal fascia and the latissimus dorsi muscle are tight.

Supine: active straight leg raise (Fig. 7.9 a,b,c)

This functional test has been investigated recently (Mens et al 1997) in a group of women suspected of having instability (impaired load transference) of the pelvic girdle. In this study, it was noted that a decreased ability to actively lift the leg in a supine position correlated highly with excessive mobility of the pelvic girdle (pubic symphysis) noted on radiography. It is proposed to be a reliable method of testing the function of the load transfer system between the spine and the leg. Clinically, it appears to be a very good screening test of function. Further

tests are necessary to differentiate the cause of the dysfunction, i.e. a breakdown in the passive or active system.

With the patient supine-lying, they are instructed to raise their leg. The ease with which they are able to do so is observed by the therapist and reported by the patient. It is also important to note any compensatory motions of the trunk during the test. When the active system is dysfunctional, the pelvic girdle will tend to rotate towards the leg which is being raised.

Subsequently, form closure can be augmented by compressing the sacroiliac joints through the innominates manually. The patient is then instructed to repeat the active straight leg raise and any change in their ability is noted and reported.

The effect of the anterior oblique system (force closure) can be assessed by asking the patient to flex and rotate the trunk towards the side of the leg to be raised. This motion is resisted manually and the patient is instructed to actively raise the leg. The difference in their ability to do so is observed and reported. The prognosis for

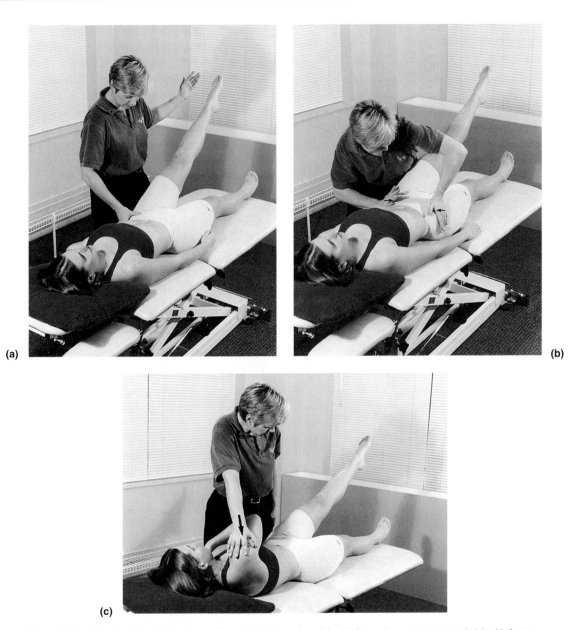

Figure 7.9   Functional test of supine-active straight leg raise; (b) with form closure augmented; (c) with force closure augmented (Mens et al 1997).

successful rehabilitation through exercise is good when an improvement in function is noted as the force closure mechanism is engaged.

Prone: active straight leg raise (Fig. 7.10a,b,c)

This functional test of integrated motor control

follows the principles of the supine active straight leg raise test. The prone patient is asked to actively extend the leg and the ability to do so is observed by the therapist and reported by the patient. The sequencing of muscle recruitment (Janda 1978) is also noted. According to Janda, the initial hamstring contraction should be

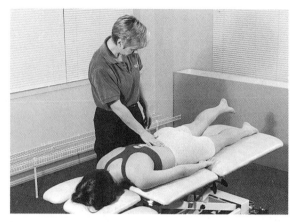

(a)

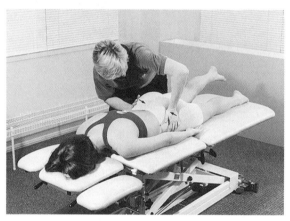

(b)

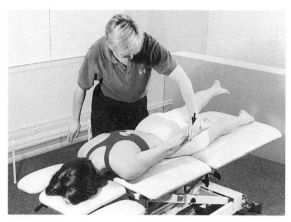

(c)

Figure 7.10 Functional test of prone-active straight leg raise; (b) with form closure augmented; (c) with force closure augmented.

followed by the ipsilateral gluteus maximus and then the contralateral erector spinae. Any excessive pelvic rotation in the transverse plane is noted. Subsequently, form closure can be augmented by compressing the sacroiliac joints through the innominates manually. The patient is then instructed to repeat the active straight leg raise and any change in their ability is noted and reported.

The effect of the posterior oblique system on the quality and ease of motion is assessed by initially recruiting the latissimus dorsi thus increasing the tension in the thoracodorsal fascia. This is done by resisting extension of the medially rotated arm prior to lifting the leg. The difference in the functional ability is observed and reported. The prognosis for successful rehabilitation through exercise is good when an improvement in function is noted as the force closure mechanism is engaged.

Articular mobility/stability tests

These tests evaluate the passive system of Panjabi's model (1992) (Fig. 5.13).

Lumbosacral junction: positional tests

When interpreting the mobility findings, the position of the joint (positional testing) at the beginning of the test should be correlated with the subsequent mobility noted, since alterations in joint mobility may merely be a reflection of an altered starting position. To determine the position of L5, the posteroanterior relationship between the transverse processes of the L5 vertebra and the sacral base is noted in full flexion and full extension. The influence of muscular hypertrophy and atrophy should be considered when interpreting the positional findings.

Flexion (Fig. 7.11). With the patient sitting, feet supported and the lumbar spine fully flexed, the L5 segment is palpated laterally with the thumbs. The posteroanterior relationship of the transverse processes of L5 relative to the sacral base is noted. A posterior right transverse process of L5 relative to the sacral base is

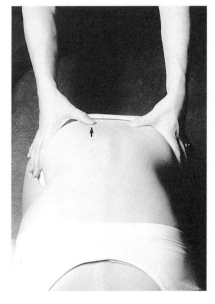

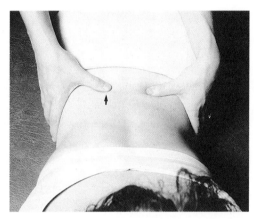

Figure 7.11

Figure 7.12

Figures 7.11 and 7.12   Positional testing of the lumbosacral junction in hyperflexion (Fig. 7.11) and in hyperextension (Fig. 7.12). Note the relative posterior position of the therapist's right thumb (arrow) when compared to the left.

indicative of a right rotated position of the L5–S1 joint complex in hyperflexion.

Extension (Fig. 7.12). With the patient prone and the lumbar spine fully extended, the L5 segment is palpated laterally with the thumbs. The posteroanterior relationship of the transverse processes of L5 relative to the sacral base is noted. A posterior right transverse process of L5 relative to the sacral base is indicative of a right rotated position of the L5–S1 joint complex in hyperextension.

Lumbosacral junction: osteokinematic tests of physiological mobility

Flexion/extension (Fig. 7.13). With the patient side-lying, hips and knees flexed and supported on the therapist's abdomen, the interspinous space between the L5 vertebra and the sacrum is palpated with the cranial hand. The caudal arm and hand supports the patient's legs above the ankles. The lumbosacral junction is passively flexed/extended and the quantity and quality of motion are noted.

Sideflexion/rotation (Fig. 7.14). With the patient

side-lying, hips and knees slightly flexed, the interspinous space between the L5 vertebra and the sacrum is palpated with the cranial hand. The caudal arm and hand palpates the pelvic girdle in an obliquely distolateral direction. The lumbosacral junction is passively sideflexed/rotated to the right and left and the quantity and quality of motion are noted.

Lumbosacral junction: arthrokinematic tests of accessory joint mobility

Superoanterior glide (Fig. 7.15). With the patient sitting, feet supported and the lumbar spine fully flexed, the transverse process of the L5 vertebra is palpated unilaterally with the thumbs. A superoanterior pressure is applied in varying directions and the quantity and end feel of motion are noted and compared to the opposite side as well as to the L4–L5 joint complex. The findings are correlated with the positional findings previously recorded.

Inferoposterior glide (Fig. 7.16). With the patient prone and the lumbar spine fully extended, the transverse process of the L5

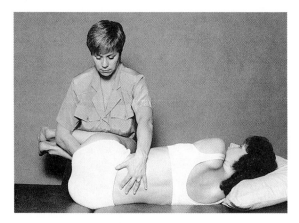

Figure 7.13 Test for passive flexion/extension of the lumbosacral junction.

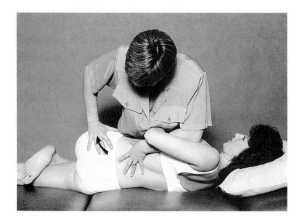

Figure 7.14 Test for passive sideflexion/rotation of the lumbosacral junction. Note the obliquity of the motion required (arrow).

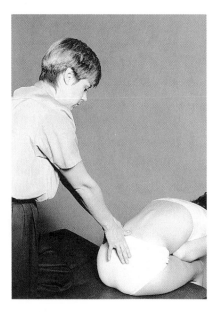

Figure 7.15 Test for passive accessory superoanterior glide at the lumbosacral junction.

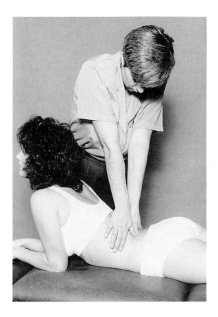

Figure 7.16 Test for passive accessory inferior glide at the lumbosacral junction.

vertebra is palpated unilaterally with the thumbs. An inferior pressure is applied in varying directions and the quantity and end feel of motion are noted and compared to the opposite side as well as to the L4–L5 joint complex. The findings are correlated with the positional findings previously recorded.

Lumbosacral junction: arthrokinetic tests of stability/stress

Compression (Fig. 7.17). This is a pain provocation or stress test, not a true stability test, since the quantity and quality of motion cannot be determined with this procedure. With the patient lying supine and the hips and knees fully flexed, the lower extremities are cradled.

Compression is applied to the vertebral column by applying a cranial force parallel to the table through the flexed lower extremities. The presence of pain and its response to compression are noted.

Torsion (Fig. 7.18). With the patient lying prone, the spinous process of the L5 vertebra is palpated with the cranial thumb. With the caudal hand, the anterior aspect of the contralateral innominate is grasped. Segmental torsion is applied by rotating the pelvis *unphysiologically* about a pure vertical axis beneath the fixed L5 vertebra (see Fig. 5.19). The joint reaction to this stress is noted both objectively (i.e. reactive muscle spasm) as well as subjectively. This test also stresses the iliolumbar ligament and the ventral sacroiliac ligament, and therefore the location of pain is not indicative of one particular structure. Stability in rotation is noted by testing axial torsion in the sidelying position. In this position, more information is gained regarding the quantity of the neutral zone and therefore an opinion can be made regarding the segment's stability.

Posteroanterior shear (Fig. 7.19). With the patient lying prone, the spinous process of the L5 vertebra is palpated with the heel of the hand. The palpating hand may be reinforced by the other for additional force. A slow, steady, posteroanterior shear is applied to the L5 vertebra. The quantity of motion (stability, neutral zone) as well as the joint reaction to this applied stress (stress test) is noted. This test may also be done in the side-lying position by fixing the spinous process of L5 and taking the pelvis posteriorly by applying compression along the flexed femurs.

Anteroposterior shear (Fig. 7.20). With the patient sitting, arms crossed, palpate the interspinous space of L5–S1. Fix the sacrum with this hand and apply a pure anteroposterior force through the trunk with the other arm/hand. Note the quantity (neutral zone) and end feel of motion (stability test) as well as the reproduction of any symptoms (stress test). This test may also be performed in full extension of L5–S1. In this position, all of the posterior translation which occurs in conjunction with extension should be

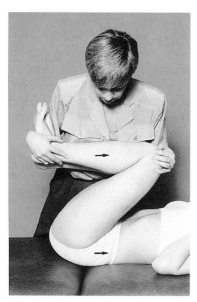

Figure 7.17

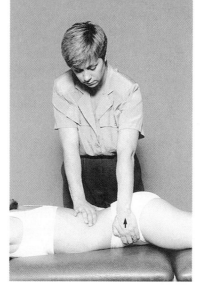

Figure 7.18

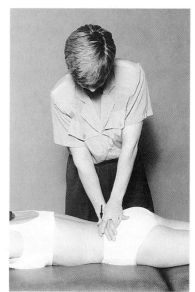

Figure 7.19

Figures 7.17, 7.18 and 7.19   Arthrokinetic tests. Compression stress test (Fig. 7.17). Torsion stress test (Fig. 7.18). Note that the rotation induced at the lumbosacral junction is about a pure vertical axis and is therefore unphysiological. Posteroanterior shear test (Fig. 7.19) for stability of the lumbosacral junction.

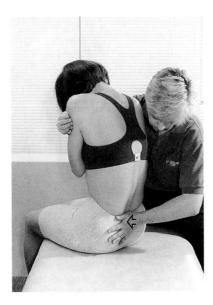

Figure 7.20 Anteroposterior shear test for stability of L5–S1.

taken up; thus no further motion should be available. When the segment is unstable in anteroposterior translation, posterior translation will still occur at the end of full extension. This is a test of passive stability. To assess the ability of the muscle system to control the excessive posterior translation, the joint is first positioned in a neutral position. The patient is then instructed to elevate their arms against the therapist's resistance and the quantity of posterior translation is palpated. When the segment is unstable passively, but stable actively, no posterior translation will occur during this test. When the segment is unstable both passively and actively, posterior translation will occur. This is a useful test of progress and can be used during stabilization training.

Pelvic girdle: positional tests

When interpreting the mobility findings, the position of the bone at the beginning of the test should be correlated with the subsequent mobility, since alterations in joint mobility may merely be a reflection of an altered starting position.

Innominate (Figs 7.21, 7.22). To determine the position of the restricted innominate, the superoinferior/mediolateral relationship of the anterior superior iliac spines, the posterior superior iliac spines and the ischial tuberosities is noted with the vertebral column in a neutral position (i.e. the patient is supine/prone). As well, the tension of the sacrotuberous ligament at its inferomedial border is assessed and correlated with the positional findings of the bones it attaches to. For example, if the innominate is posteriorly rotated, the sacrotuberous ligament should be taut since the points of attachment are attenuated. However, if the innominate is anteriorly rotated, the sacrotuberous ligament should be relatively slack since the points of attachment are approximated.

Sacrum (Fig. 7.23). Positional testing of the sacrum should be evaluated in three positions of the trunk: flexion, extension and neutral. In flexion, the sacral position is assessed with the patient sitting, feet supported and the lumbar spine fully flexed. The patient is prone for evaluation in neutral and prone in full lumbar extension for evaluation in extension. To determine the position of the sacrum, a comparison is made of the posteroanterior relationship of the inferior lateral angle bilaterally and the posteroanterior relationship of the sacral base bilaterally. An anterior right sacral base together with a posterior left inferior lateral angle is indicative of a left rotated sacrum. An anterior left sacral base together with a posterior right inferior lateral angle is indicative of a right rotated sacrum. In isolation, these findings are not diagnostic of any particular dysfunction. They must be correlated with mobility findings in the lumbosacral, sacroiliac and hip joints for their significance to be understood.

Pelvic girdle: arthrokinematic tests of accessory joint mobility

Inferoposterior glide innominate/sacrum (Fig. 7.24). (Lee 1992, Lee & Walsh 1996). With the long and ring finger of one hand, palpate the

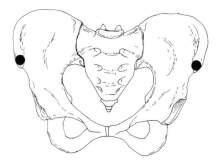

Figure 7.21 Points of anterior palpation for positional testing of the innominate.

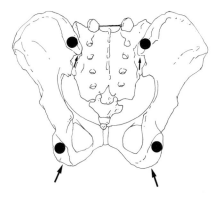

Figure 7.22 Points of posterior palpation (large arrows) for positional testing of the innominate. The inferior aspect (small arrows) of the PSIS and the ischial tuberosity (dots) are palpated bilaterally and the superoinferior/mediolateral relationship noted.

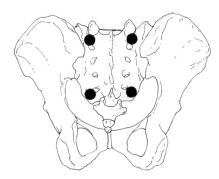

Figure 7.23 Points of palpation for positional testing of the sacrum.

sacral sulcus just medial to the PSIS (Fig. 7.25). With the index finger of the same hand, palpate the lumbosacral junction. The long and ring

Mobility Tests Innominate/Sacrum

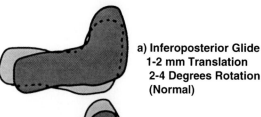
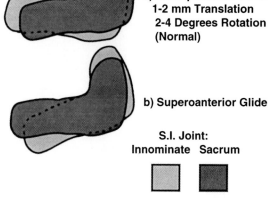

a) Inferoposterior Glide
1-2 mm Translation
2-4 Degrees Rotation
(Normal)

b) Superoanterior Glide

S.I. Joint:
Innominate Sacrum

Figure 7.24 Exaggerated illustration of the direction of joint glides tested in the arthrokinematic tests of sacroiliac (S.I.) joint mobility.

finger monitor motion between the innominate and the sacrum, while the index finger notes any movement between the pelvic girdle and the L5 vertebra. With the heel of the other hand, palpate the ipsilateral ASIS and the iliac crest. Apply an anterior rotation force (Fig. 7.26) to the innominate to produce an inferoposterior glide at the sacroiliac joint. Note the quantity, direction of ease and the end feel of motion. This glide is also associated with counternutation of the sacrum. The end of the range of motion is reached when the pelvic girdle is felt to rotate as a unit beneath the L5 vertebra.

Superoanterior glide innominate/sacrum (Fig. 7.27) (Lee 1992, Lee & Walsh 1996). With the long and ring finger of one hand, palpate the sacral sulcus just medial to the PSIS (Fig. 7.25). With the index finger of the same hand, palpate the lumbosacral junction. The long and ring finger monitor motion between the innominate and the sacrum, while the index finger notes any movement between the pelvic girdle and the L5 vertebra. With the heel of the other hand, palpate the ipsilateral ASIS and the iliac crest. Apply a posterior rotation force (Fig. 7.27) to the innominate to produce a superoanterior glide at the sacroiliac joint. Note the quantity, direction

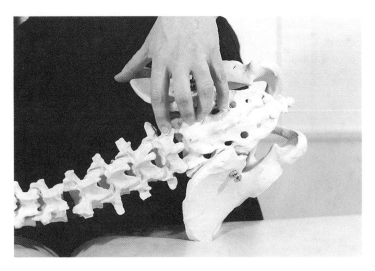

Figure 7.25   Position of the posterior hand for palpation during mobility and stability testing of the sacroiliac joint.

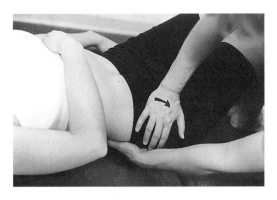

Figure 7.26   Anterior rotation of the innominate requires an inferoposterior glide at the sacroiliac joint.

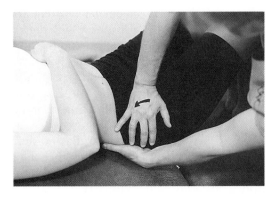

Figure 7.27   Posterior rotation of the innominate requires a superoanterior glide at the sacroiliac joint.

of ease and the end feel of motion. This glide is also associated with nutation of the sacrum. The end of the range of motion is reached when the pelvic girdle is felt to rotate as a unit beneath the L5 vertebra.

Pelvic girdle: arthrokinetic tests of stability

These tests are used to detect a change in the neutral zone of the sacroiliac joint (Fig. 7.28a). They specifically evaluate the ability of the joint to resist vertical and horizontal plane translation (Lee 1992, 1997b, Lee & Walsh 1996). When there has been severe damage to the ligamentous structures of the sacroiliac joint, the neutral zone is increased (Panjabi 1992) (Fig. 7.28b). In this situation, there is a softer end feel of motion, an increased quantity of translation and a variable symptom response. If the joint is irritable, the test may provoke pain and subsequently muscle spasm; however pain is not a criterion for biomechanical diagnoses. If the instability is long standing and asymptomatic, the tests are often not provocative.

If the sacroiliac joint has been previously sprained and the capsule has become fibrosed, the neutral zone is decreased but a glide or joint play is still available (Fig. 7.28c). The quantity of

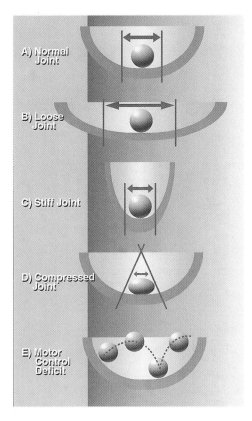

Figure 7.28 **(a)** A graphic illustration of motion in a normal neutral zone (Redrawn from Panjabi 1992). **(b)** When form closure is lost, motion within the neutral zone is increased. **(c)** When the joint is fibrosed, motion in the neutral zone is decreased. **(d)** When there are excessive compressive forces across the joint, motion within the neutral zone is completely blocked. **(e)** When there is a motor control deficit, *passive* motion within the neutral zone is normal since the dysfunction is dynamic. Functionally, as the ball moves in the bowl, approximation is intermittently lost and then regained.

dynamic. A graphic respresentation of this condition is illustrated in Figure 7.28e.

Anteroposterior translation: innominate/sacrum (Fig. 7.29). With the patient supine and the knees and hips flexed, the sacral sulcus just medial to the PSIS is palpated with the long and ring fingers while the index finger of this hand palpates the lumbosacral junction (Fig. 7.25). The long and ring fingers monitor translation between the innominate and the sacrum while the index finger notes any movement between the pelvic girdle and the L5 vertebra.

A posterior pressure is applied to the innominate through the iliac crest and the ASIS (Fig. 7.30) and the relative mobility is noted posteriorly. The end of the range of motion is reached when the pelvic girdle rotates as a unit beneath the L5 vertebra. The motion is

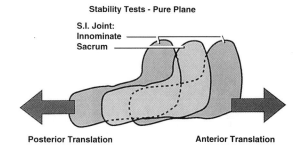

Figure 7.29 Posteroanterior and anteroposterior translation tests examine the ability of the sacroiliac joint to resist horizontal translation forces.

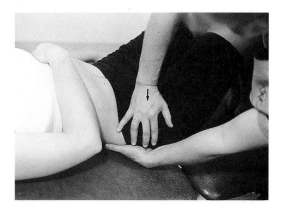

Figure 7.30 A posterior translation force is applied to the innominate and the motion is noted posteriorly.

motion is reduced and the end feel is hard. If the transarticular muscles are overactive, compression of the sacroiliac joint is excessive and these tests will reveal minimal, if any, motion available (Fig. 7.28d).

There is another situation in which the neutral zone is normal but there is insufficient motor control, or appropriate timing of muscle contraction, to maintain sufficient articular compression throughout the motion. This dysfunction is not apparent on passive testing of joint play since the impaired load transfer is compared to that on the opposite side. The quality of the end feel, the quantity of translation and the reproduction of any symptoms are noted.

Superoinferior translation: innominate/sacrum (Fig. 7.31). To test superoinferior translation, a superior/inferior pressure is applied to the innominate through the distal end of the femur or through the ischial tuberosity. The relative mobility is noted posteriorly (Fig. 7.32). The end of the range of motion is reached when the pelvic girdle is felt to bend laterally beneath the L5 vertebra. The motion is compared to that on the opposite side. The quality of the end feel, the quantity of translation and the reproduction of any symptoms are noted.

Superoinferior translation: pubic symphysis (Fig. 7.33) (Lee & Walsh 1996). With the heel of one hand, palpate the superior aspect of the superior ramus of one pubic bone. With the heel of the other hand, palpate the inferior aspect of the superior ramus of the opposite pubic bone. Fix one pubic bone and apply a slow, steady inferosuperior force to the other and note the quantity and the end feel of motion as well as the reproduction of any symptoms. Switch hands and repeat the test such that each side is stressed superiorly and inferiorly.

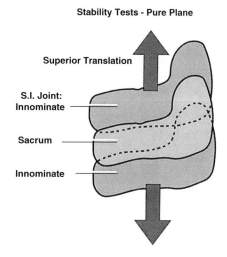

Stability Tests - Pure Plane

Superior Translation

S.I. Joint: Innominate

Sacrum

Innominate

Figure 7.31 Superoinferior translation tests examine the ability of the sacroiliac joint to resist vertical translation forces.

Pain provocation tests

Pain provocation tests have shown good inter-tester reliability (Laslett 1994, 1997) although their validity and specificity have been questioned (Dreyfuss et al 1994, 1996). They are useful if injection therapy is going to be part of the treatment plan (Gillies & Griesdale 1997).

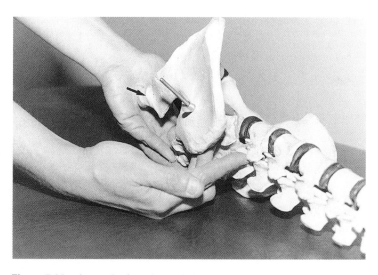

Figure 7.32 A superior force is applied to the innominate and the motion is noted posteriorly.

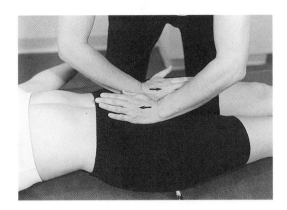

Figure 7.33 Superoinferior translation test for the pubic symphysis.

Transverse anterior distraction–posterior compression (Fig. 7.34) (Lee & Walsh 1996). With the patient lying supine, the medial aspect of the anterior superior iliac spine is palpated bilaterally with the heels of the crossed hands. A slow, steady, posterolateral force is applied through the pelvic girdle, thus distracting the ventral aspect of the sacroiliac joint and pubic symphysis and compressing the posterior structures. The force is maintained for 20 seconds and the provocation and location of pain is noted. The ventral sacroiliac ligament can be palpated at Baer's point located approximately 2.5 cm medial to the ASIS deep within the pelvis. Exquisite tenderness at this point is indicative of

either an irritable ligament and/or iliacus muscle spasm.

Transverse posterior distraction–anterior compression (Fig. 7.35) (Lee & Walsh 1996). With the patient side-lying, hips and knees comfortably flexed, the anterolateral aspect of the uppermost iliac crest is palpated. A slow, steady, medial force is applied through the pelvic girdle, thus distracting the posterior structures of the sacroiliac joint and compressing the anterior. The force is maintained for 20 seconds and the provocation and location of pain is noted.

Long dorsal sacroiliac ligament (Fig. 7.36) (Lee & Walsh 1996). With the patient prone, palpate the sacral apex in the midline with one hand. Reinforce this hand with the other. Apply an anterior force to the sacrum thus forcing the sacrum to counternutate. The force is maintained for 20 seconds and the provocation and location of pain is noted.

Sacrotuberous/interosseous ligaments (Fig. 7.37) (Lee & Walsh 1996). With the patient prone, palpate the sacral base in the midline with one hand. Reinforce this hand with the other. Apply an anterior force to the sacrum thus forcing the

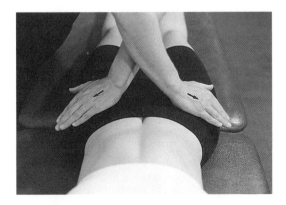

Figure 7.34 This pain provocation test stresses the anterior structures of the pelvic girdle and compresses those posterior.

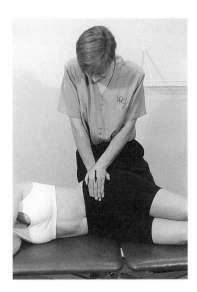

Figure 7.35 This pain provocation test stresses the posterior structures of the pelvic girdle and compresses those anterior.

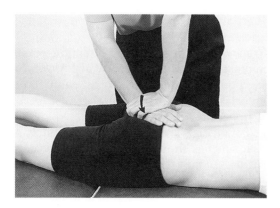

Figure 7.36 This pain provocation test stresses the long dorsal sacroiliac ligament.

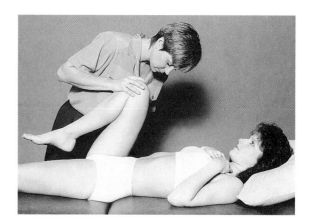

Figure 7.38 Test for passive flexion of the femur at the hip joint.

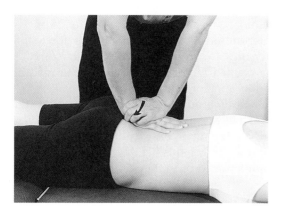

Figure 7.37 This pain provocation test stresses the sacrotuberous and interosseous ligaments.

Both the quantity of motion as well as the end feel are noted. The test is repeated on and compared to the opposite side.

Extension (Fig. 7.39). With the patient supine, lying at the end of the table, one femur is fully flexed against the trunk, held by the patient and supported against the therapist's lateral thorax. The anterior aspect of the iliac crest and the anterior superior iliac spine of the limb being

sacrum to nutate. The force is maintained for 20 seconds and the provocation and location of pain is noted.

Hip: osteokinematic tests of physiological mobility

Flexion (Fig. 7.38). With the patient lying supine, the flexed knee of the lower extremity to be tested is palpated with the caudal hand. The anterior aspect of the iliac crest and the anterior superior iliac spine are palpated with the cranial hand. The femur is passively flexed at the hip joint until posterior rotation of the ipsilateral innominate begins. At that point, the limit of available range for femoral flexion has occurred.

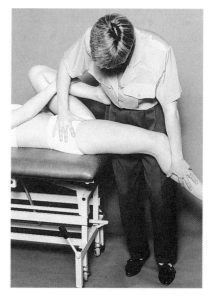

Figure 7.39 Test for passive extension of the femur at the hip joint.

tested are palpated with the cranial hand. With the caudal hand, the therapist guides the femur into extension until anterior rotation of the ipsilateral innominate begins. At that point, the limit of available range for femoral extension has occurred. Both the quantity of motion as well as the end feel are noted. The test is repeated on and compared to the opposite side.

Abduction/adduction (Fig. 7.40). With the patient supine, lying at the end of the table, one femur is fully flexed against the trunk, held by the patient and supported against the therapist's lateral thorax. The anterior aspect of the iliac crest and the anterior superior iliac spine of the limb being tested are palpated with the cranial hand. With the caudal hand, the therapist guides the femur into abduction/adduction until lateral bending of the pelvic girdle beneath the vertebral column begins. At that point, the limit of femoral abduction/adduction has been reached. Both the quantity of motion as well as the end feel are noted. The test is repeated on and compared to the opposite side.

Lateral/medial rotation (Fig. 7.41). With the patient lying supine, the lower extremity to be tested is palpated above the ankle with the caudal hand. The test can be performed in varying degrees of hip flexion/extension to assist in the differentiation between an articular and myofascial restriction. The anterior aspect of the iliac crest and the anterior superior iliac spine

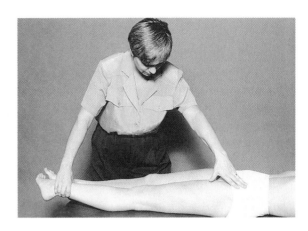

Figure 7.41   Test for passive medial rotation of the femur at the hip joint in neutral.

are palpated with the cranial hand. The femur is passively laterally/medially rotated until rotation of the innominate begins. At that point, the limit of available range for femoral rotation has occurred. Both the quantity of motion as well as the end feel are noted. The test is repeated on and compared to the opposite side.

Quadrant test (Fig. 7.42). With the patient lying supine, the flexed knee of the lower extremity to be tested is palpated with the caudal hand. The anterior aspect of the iliac crest and the anterior superior iliac spine are palpated with the cranial

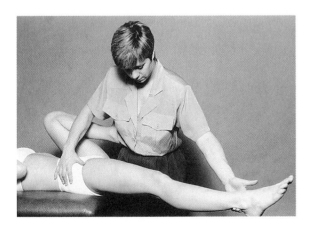

Figure 7.40   Test for passive abduction of the femur at the hip joint.

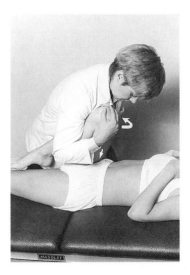

Figure 7.42   Quadrant test of the hip joint.

hand. The femur is passively flexed, adducted, medially rotated and longitudinally compressed to scour the inner aspect of the joint. From this position, the femur is taken into abduction and lateral rotation while maintaining the degree of femoral flexion and longitudinal compression. Both the quality of motion and the presence/location of pain are noted. The test is repeated on and compared to the opposite extremity.

Hip: arthrokinematic tests of accessory joint mobility

Motions of linear translation are relatively limited at the hip joint in comparison to angular motions. Consequently, movement analysis of linear translation will be less informative than analysis of the physiological motions.

Lateral/medial translation (Fig. 7.43). With the patient lying supine and the femur flexed to 30° (resting position of the hip joint), the proximal thigh is palpated. The joint is translated laterally by applying an inferolateral force parallel to the neck of the femur. The motion has been termed lateral translation, in keeping with Fig. 5.12. The superior and inferior aspects of the head of the femur translate laterally in relation to the acetabulum while the fovea is distracted. Medial translation is applied by approximating the femur superomedially into the medial aspect of the acetabular fossa. The quantity of motion, the end feel and the presence/location of pain are noted.

Distraction/compression (Fig. 7.44). With the patient lying supine and the femur flexed to 30°, the proximal thigh is palpated. The superior aspect of the joint is distracted by applying an inferior force along the longitudinal axis of the femur. Compression is applied by approximating the femur superiorly into the superior aspect of the acetabular fossa. The quantity of motion, the end feel and the presence/location of pain are noted.

Anteroposterior/posteroanterior glide (Fig. 7.45). With the patient lying supine and the femur flexed to 30°, the proximal thigh is palpated. An anteroposterior glide is induced by applying a posterolateral force perpendicular to the line of the femoral neck. A posteroanterior glide is induced by applying an anteromedial force perpendicular to the line of the femoral

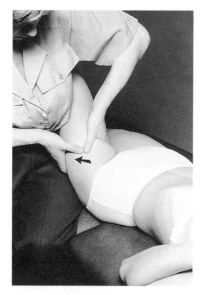
Figure 7.43

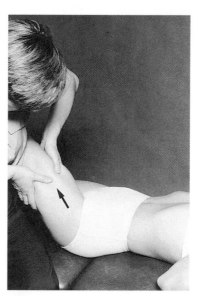
Figure 7.44

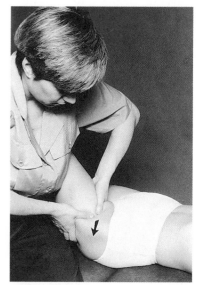
Figure 7.45

Figures 7.43, 7.44 and 7.45 Arthrokinematic tests at the hip: for lateral translation, distraction and anteroposterior glide.

neck. The quantity of motion, the end feel and the presence/location of pain are noted.

Hip: arthrokinetic tests of stability

Proprioception/arthrokinetic stability (Fig. 7.46). This is a useful test of integrated neuro-muscular function (see Ch. 4, Microscopic articular neurology) of the weight-bearing lumbo-pelvic-hip region. With the patient standing in front of a plumb-line, he/she is instructed to bear weight unilaterally without support and to subsequently close their eyes. The degree of lateral shift of the center of gravity from the plumb-line is observed and compared to the opposite side.

Torque test (Fig. 7.47). This is a global test of passive stability and a pain provocation test for the ligaments of the hip joint. The intent is to stress all of the capsular ligaments simultaneously. If the test is painless, then the subsequent tests, which help to differentiate the individual ligaments, are not required.

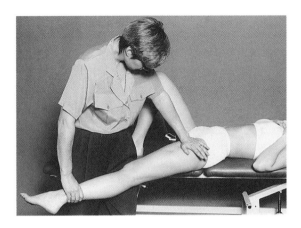

Figure 7.47 The torque test is a global test of passive stability and a pain provocation test for the ligaments of the hip joint.

With the patient supine, lying close to the edge of the table, the ipsilateral femur is extended until anterior rotation of the innominate begins. The femur is then medially rotated to the limit of the physiological range of motion. The proximal thigh is palpated and a slow, steady, postero-lateral force is applied along the line of the neck of the femur to further stress the capsular ligaments. The force is maintained for 20 seconds and the quality of the end feel and the provocation of local pain is noted.

Inferior band of the iliofemoral ligament. This ligament is taut when the femur is fully extended. If passive femoral extension elicits the greatest amount of pain, this ligament may be the etiological factor.

Iliotrochanteric band of the iliofemoral ligament. With the patient supine, lying close to the edge of the table, the ipsilateral femur is slightly extended, *adducted* and fully laterally rotated. The distal femur is fixed against the therapist's thigh and the proximal femur is palpated. A slow, steady, posterolateral force is applied along the line of the neck of the femur and the provocation of local pain is noted.

Pubofemoral ligament (Fig. 7.48). With the patient lying supine, the ipsilateral femur is slightly extended, *abducted* and fully laterally rotated. The distal femur is fixed against the therapist's thigh and the proximal femur is

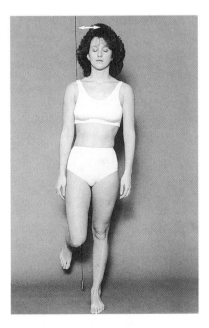

Figure 7.46 Weight-bearing test of proprioception of weight transfer in the lumbo-pelvic-hip region. Note the degree of lateral shift of the center of gravity from the plumb-line (arrow).

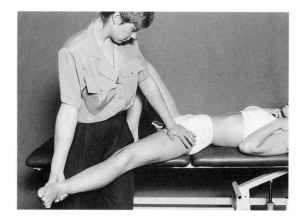

Figure 7.48 Pubofemoral ligament stress test.

palpated. A slow, steady, posterolateral force is applied along the line of the neck of the femur and the provocation of local pain is noted.

Ischiofemoral ligament. With the patient lying supine, the ipsilateral femur is slightly extended, abducted and fully *medially* rotated. The distal femur is fixed against the therapist's thigh and the proximal femur is palpated. A slow, steady, anterolateral force is applied along the line of the neck of the femur and the provocation of local pain is noted.

Muscle function tests

These tests evaluate the active system of Panjabi's model (1992) (Fig. 5.13), the force closure mechanism. Dysfunction of the active system is noted initially during the functional tests. Subsequently, the ability of the patient to isolate and sustain a contraction of a specific muscle of the inner or outer unit is examined. The biomechanics of the force closure mechanism have been previously described in Chapter 5. It is not the intent of this section to duplicate the complete work of Kendall et al (1993) whose text is highly recommended for further discussion on specific muscle testing. The intention is to show how specific muscle testing can be used to identify the components of the force closure mechanism (inner unit vs. outer unit) which are in dysfunction so that exercise programs may be developed in accordance with

the biomechanical model. When this approach is used, evidence-based rehabilitation can be practised and tested through future research.

Muscle recruitment/strength: force closure

The following tests evaluate the ability of the patient to isolate and sustain a specific contraction of the inner and/or outer unit muscles and then to maintain control (force closure mechanism) of the lumbar spine and pelvic girdle under increasing loads. Myofascial stability requires adequate strength and appropriate timing during functional tasks.

Inner unit: transversus abdominis/multifidus/ levator ani. In patients with chronic low back pain, it has been shown (Richardson & Jull 1994) that at low load levels, endurance rather than strength is the main deficit. The tests therefore must involve an isometric contraction for a set period of time (10 seconds). When in dysfunction, a muscle may display an inability to sustain a hold or produce a more phasic, jerky pattern of contraction when the hold is sustained. These tests determine the ability of the patient to isolate a holding contraction of the inner unit (transversus abdominis, multifidus and the pelvic floor) under increasing levels of load.

To test for isolation of the transversus abdominis, the patient is prone and a pressure biofeedback unit (Richardson & Jull 1994, 1995) is placed underneath the abdomen (Fig. 7.49). The cuff is inflated to a base level of 70 mmHg. The patient is instructed to draw the navel up and in towards the chest (abdominal hollowing). The abdomen can be palpated 2 cm medial and inferior to the ASIS to ensure the appropriate contraction of the transversus abdominis (Hodges 1997c). At this point, the transversus abdominis is approximately 4 mm thick and the internal oblique is 15 mm thick. When the transversus abdominis contracts, an increase in tension, not bulging, is felt at the point noted above. When the internal oblique contracts, a distinct bulging is felt (Hodges 1997c).

The multifidus muscle is also palpated to ensure its co-contraction with the transversus abdominis. The appropriate tonic response is a

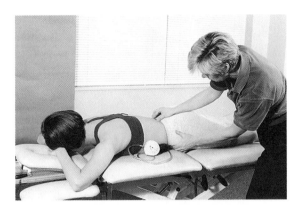

Figure 7.49 Testing position for isolation of the inner unit. The lower abdomen and the multifidus are palpated to ensure their appropriate contraction.

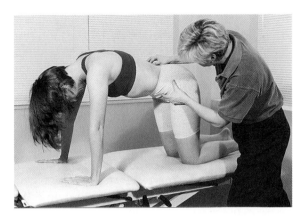

Figure 7.50 An alternative position for testing isolation of the inner unit. When the transversus abdominis contracts correctly, the lower abdomen elevates before the upper abdomen and the lateral costal margin remains still.

slow, steady swelling of the muscle just lateral to the spinous process. An inappropriate, phasic response is quick and short lasting (Hodges 1997c).

During this test, any substitution strategies by the rectus abdominis (posterior pelvic tilt) and the oblique abdominals (in- or out-flaring of the lower lateral costal margins) are observed and the pressure change in the biofeedback cuff is noted. When the transversus abdominis is recruited in isolation, the pressure should drop 6–8 mmHg. Large pressure decreases indicate that the patient is using the rectus abdominis to flex the lumbar spine. Pressure increases indicate that the lumbar lordosis is increasing and that the neutral spinal position has been lost.

When the multifidus is weak or atrophied, a palpable dip can be felt just lateral to the spinous process of the affected segment. When the patient is asked to 'swell' the multifidus muscle (Richardson & Jull 1995) the lack of recruitment can be felt locally.

Alternatively, isolation of the transversus abdominis and multifidus can be tested in the four-point kneeling position (Fig. 7.50). To begin, the patient's shoulders and hips are centered over the hands and knees and the lumbar spine is in a neutral position. From this position, the patient is instructed to completely relax the abdomen. The transversus abdominis is isolated by having the patient take a breath in, breathe out and then draw the navel up towards the spine (abdominal hollowing) (Hodges 1997c, Richardson & Jull 1995). When done properly, the lower abdomen should elevate before the upper abdomen and the oblique muscles should remain relaxed. The lower rib cage should not expand nor contract.

The multifidus is isolated in this position by palpating the muscle lateral to the spinous process or directly over the dorsum of the sacrum. To test the patient's ability to isolate the multifidus, the instruction is to make the muscle harden or swell under the therapist's fingers.

Physiotherapists who specialize in urinary and anorectal dysfunction routinely use intra-vaginal tests to evaluate the strength and timing of contraction of the four pelvic floor muscles. This is probably the best way to evaluate this region. Recent study (Sapsford et al 1998) has suggested that there is an inter-relationship between the abdominal wall and the muscles of the pelvic floor (Ch. 5). This relationship can be tested by musculoskeletal therapists who choose not to use internal examination techniques, although the information gained will not be as specific. Collectively, all four parts of the levator ani muscle counternutate the sacrum. Although the pelvic floor does not work in isolation from the abdominal wall, patients who are able to isolate this component of the inner unit are able to counternutate the sacrum without any motion occurring between the pelvic girdle and the femur or the pelvic girdle and the lumbar spine. To test the functional inter-relationship and the ability of the patient to recruit the pelvic floor collectively, the patient is supine with hips and knees flexed. The therapist palpates the sacral apex dorsally and the abdominal wall 2 cm medial and inferior to the ASIS. The patient is instructed to shorten the distance between coccyx and pubic symphysis (an anatomy lesson precedes this instruction), thus drawing the muscles of the pelvic floor internally. When done appropriately, the sacrum will counternutate (apex moves away from your hand) and the transversus abdominis will be felt to contract (tension will be increased at the point 2 cm medial and inferior to the ASIS; the abdomen should not bulge at this point). Sapsford feels (personal communication) that it is possible to retrain the various muscles of the pelvic floor using the abdominals. She suggests that isolation of the transversus abdominis facilitates the co-contraction of the pubococcygeus whereas the obliques facilitate the ilio- and ischiococcygeus. This hypothesis remains to be scientifically tested. If the patient is unable to isolate a contraction of the pelvic floor within 2 weeks of exercise instruction, a referral to a physio-therapist who specializes in pelvic floor dysfunction is indicated.

If the patient is able to isolate the muscles of the inner unit appropriately, the test is made more difficult by increasing the load. With the patient supine, the hips and knees are flexed and the pressure biofeedback unit is placed beneath the lumbar spine. The cuff is inflated to a base level of 40 mmHg and the patient is asked to 'hollow the abdomen'. The ability to do so is noted as in the prone test. The pressure should increase no more than 10–15 mmHg. Loads are increased through the upper and lower extremity in a progressive manner, increasing both the weight and the lever arm (Fig. 7.51). A static holding test is advocated by Richardson & Jull (1994, 1995) because these muscles are required to contract for prolonged periods of time during stabilization of the spine and pelvic

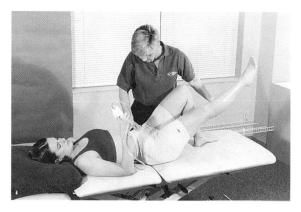

Figure 7.51   The ability to maintain a neutral lumbar spine under increasing loads is evaluated with a pressure biofeedback unit (Richardson & Jull 1994, 1995).

girdle. The patient should be able to sustain a 10-second hold repeated 10 times without losing a neutral lumbar spine position.

Outer unit: posterior oblique, anterior oblique, lateral systems. The posterior oblique system consists of the gluteus maximus and latissimus dorsi muscles and the intervening thoracodorsal fascia. When the gluteus maximus is weak, the buttock appears flattened and the gluteal fold may be lower on the weak side in standing.

The gluteus maximus is specifically tested in the prone position (Kendall et al 1993). The patient is asked to squeeze the buttocks together and the ability to do so is palpated. If the patient is able to isolate an effective contraction, they are then asked to perform a concentric contraction by extending the femur with the knee flexed (Fig. 7.52). Resistance is then applied to the extended femur. Careful observation of the effects of this contraction on the position of the lumbar spine gives the examiner further information on the ability of the patient to stabilize effectively. It is not uncommon to find positional weakness of the gluteus maximus muscle in patients with a chronically anteriorly rotated innominate. This position lengthens the gluteus maximus muscle and when this muscle is tested in its shortened position, a marked weakness will be found.

The latissimus dorsi is isolated by resisting adduction of the extended, medially rotated arm

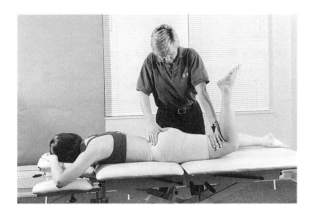

Figure 7.52 Concentric contraction of gluteus maximus in a shortened position. This muscle often tests weak in the presence of an anteriorly rotated innominate.

(Fig. 7.53). This muscle tends to tighten along with the thoracodorsal fascia and its length has been tested in the functional tests.

The anterior oblique system consists of the oblique abdominals and the contralateral adductors of the thigh. When the anterior system is weak, the abdomen tends to protrude and the pelvic girdle to anteriorly rotate on the femoral heads in standing. The obliques are isolated in the crook lying position. The patient is instructed to brace (not hollow) their abdomen thereby expanding their waist laterally. When the external obliques are recruited in isolation, the infrasternal angle will narrow and the lateral costal margin will be compressed. When the

internal obliques are recruited in isolation, the infrasternal angle will widen and the lateral costal margin will expand. In the braced position with both the external and internal obliques recruited, most patients will also recruit their rectus abdominis isometrically. This collective contraction should result in a reflex tightening of all of the muscles of the pelvic floor (Sapsford et al 1998).

The lateral system consists of the gluteus medius/minimus and the adductors of the thigh. The ability to isolate a contraction of the anterior fibers of gluteus medius is tested according to Kendall et al (1993) (Fig. 7.54). The patient is side-lying with the leg to be tested uppermost. With the knee extended, the leg is positioned in slight extension, abduction and internal rotation. The patient is requested to hold the trunk and the leg still, as support is released. The response is then observed. The patient with weak anterior fibers of gluteus medius will tend to rotate the pelvis backwards to facilitate the use of the tensor fascia lata. Alternatively, they may sideflex the spine in an attempt to hold the leg. In both cases, stabilization of the lumbar spine has been lost in an attempt to achieve the task demanded. If the patient can hold the proper trunk and leg position for 10 seconds, resistance is applied to the leg into flexion, adduction and external rotation. When the anterior fibers of gluteus

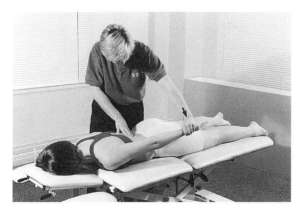

Figure 7.53 Isolation of latissimus dorsi.

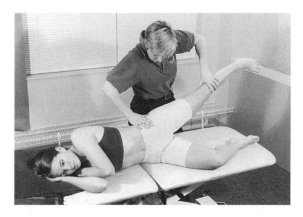

Figure 7.54 Isolation of the anterior fibers of the gluteus medius (Kendall et al 1993).

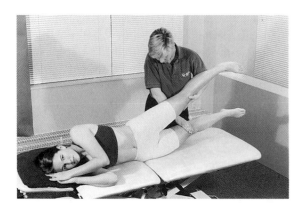

Figure 7.55 Isolation of the adductors of the thigh.

medius are weak, the leg gives easily. In addition, atrophy of the upper lateral quadrant of the buttock can be seen and felt.

The posterior fibers of gluteus medius are also tested in side-lying. The hips and knees are slightly flexed. The patient is instructed to maintain contact between the ankles and then to lift the top knee (externally rotate the hip). Resistance to external rotation is applied through the lateral aspect of the femur. When the posterior fibers of gluteus medius are weak, the leg gives way easily and the patient attempts to compensate by rotating the pelvis backwards to facilitate the use of the tensor fascia lata. Alternatively, they may sideflex the spine in an attempt to hold the leg.

The adductors are isolated by having the patient adduct the bottom leg while the therapist holds the upper leg in abduction (Fig. 7.55). Careful observation of stabilization of the trunk during this test yields further information on motor control.

Muscle length

Muscle shortening can adversely affect the biomechanics of the lumbo-pelvic-hip region (Ch. 5). The muscles which tend to tighten in the presence of dysfunction (Janda 1986) should be assessed for their extensibility. These muscles include erector spinae, hamstrings, rectus femoris, iliopsoas, tensor fascia lata, adductors, and piriformis. A functional test for the length of

the latissimus dorsi and the thoracodorsal fascia has been discussed.

Erector spinae. With the patient sitting, feet supported and the vertebral column in a neutral position, the patient is instructed to forward bend. The quantity of the available motion, the symmetry/asymmetry of the paravertebral muscles and the presence/absence of a multisegmental spinal curve at the limit of range are noted. A multisegmental rotoscoliosis may be indicative of unilateral tightness of the erector spinae muscles.

Hamstrings (semimembranosus, semitendinosus, biceps femoris). Dysfunction of this muscle group is first revealed in the functional sitting test. Specific examination of hamstring extensibility is performed with the patient lying supine and the lower extremity to be tested flexed at the hip joint to 90°. While maintaining the femur in this position, the knee is extended until the first resistance from the hamstrings is encountered (Fig. 7.56). Medial and lateral rotation of the femur will bias the test towards the medial or lateral hamstring. Both the quantity and the end feel of motion are noted. The test is repeated on and compared to the opposite extremity.

What is normal length? According to Kendall et al (1993), when hamstring length is measured with the lumbar spine in a neutral position and no motion of the pelvic girdle allowed, the femur

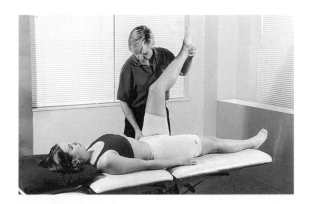

Figure 7.56 Test for hamstring length. The test can be biased towards the biceps femoris by laterally rotating the femur and towards the medial hamstring group by medially rotating the femur.

should flex at the hip joint to 70°. Clinically, one needs to consider the patient's functional demands. This quantity of motion would be insufficient for a dancer or for a person who works in repetitive trunk flexion or who drives a car with a low seat. If the patient presents with lumbo-pelvic-hip *pain* and the pain provocation tests have revealed that the pelvic ligaments are a potential source of this pain, then the hamstrings need to be extensible enough to allow full forward bending with counternutation of the sacrum occurring only at the very end of the motion (see pelvic girdle, active physiological mobility tests, Fig. 7.4).

Iliopsoas, rectus femoris, anterior band tensor fascia lata, adductors (Figs 7.57, 7.58, 7.59). With the patient supine, lying at the end of the table, one femur is flexed until the lumbar spine is in a neutral position. The knee is held by the patient and supported against the therapist's lateral thorax. The anterior aspect of the iliac crest and the anterior superior iliac spine of the limb being tested are palpated. With the other hand, the therapist guides the femur into extension with the knee extended to test the length of the

iliopsoas muscle and then with the knee flexed to test the length of the rectus femoris muscle. Both the quantity of femoral extension and knee flexion as well as the end feel of motion are noted. The test is repeated on and compared to the opposite extremity.

An inextensible iliopsoas muscle will restrict extension of the femur regardless of the position of the knee whereas an inextensible rectus femoris muscle will only restrict extension of the femur if the knee is flexed. According to Kendall et al (1993), in this position, the thigh should reach the table and the knee should flex to 80°.

If the anterior band of the tensor fascia lata muscle is tight, full femoral extension will occur only if the hip is allowed to abduct. In addition, knee flexion with femoral extension results in lateral tibial rotation when the muscle is tight. If the tibial rotation is passively blocked during the test, knee flexion will be restricted.

The length of the adductors is tested with femoral abduction. The short adductors are tested with the knee flexed, the long adductors with the knee extended. Both the quantity and the end feel of motion are noted. The test is

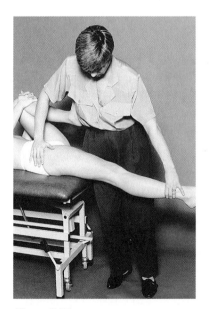 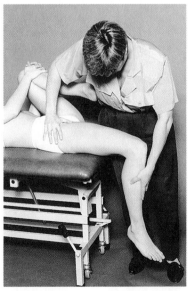 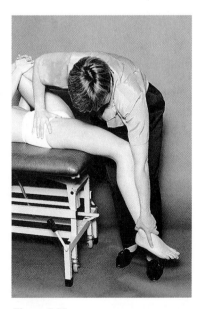

Figure 7.57   **Figure 7.58**   **Figure 7.59**

Figures 7.57, 7.58 and 7.59 Tests for extensibility of the iliopsoas muscle, the rectus femoris muscle and the anterior band of the tensor fascia lata muscle.

repeated on and compared to the opposite extremity.

Middle band of tensor fascia lata (Kendall et al 1993) (Fig. 7.60). With the patient side-lying and the bottom limb comfortably flexed, the anteromedial aspect of the femur is grasped with the caudal hand and the extended knee supported by the therapist's caudal hand and forearm. The pelvic girdle is supported with the cranial hand while the caudal hand flexes, abducts and then extends the femur to neutral or into slight extension. The femur is then guided into adduction. Both the quantity of femoral adduction and the quality of the end feel are noted. The test is repeated on and compared to the opposite extremity. An inextensible tensor fascia lata muscle will restrict femoral adduction and often produces a lateral patellar tilt during this test. Both the quantity and the end feel of motion are noted. The test is repeated on and compared to the opposite extremity.

Piriformis (Fig. 7.61). The patient is supine, the lower extremity comfortably flexed at the hip and knee. The lateral aspect of the iliac crest and the anterior superior iliac spine are palpated with the cranial hand, while the caudal hand flexes the femur to 60° of flexion. At this point, the piriformis muscle acts as a pure abductor of the femur (Kapandji 1974). Before 60° it also laterally rotates the femur, while after 60° it medially rotates the femur. From 60° of femoral flexion, the femur is guided into adduction with

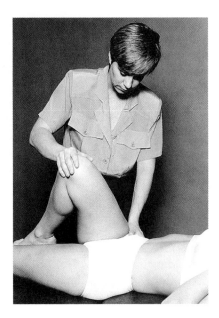

Figure 7.61   Test for extensibility of the piriformis muscle. At 60° of femoral flexion, this muscle acts as a pure femoral abductor.

the caudal hand while the cranial hand monitors the subsequent medial rotation of the innominate. The extensibility of the piriformis muscle has been reached when the innominate is felt to medially rotate. If the femur is taken beyond 60° of flexion, lateral femoral rotation is required to fully stretch the muscle. Both the quantity and the end feel of motion are noted. The test is repeated on and compared to the opposite extremity.

Contractile lesions

The tests for muscle function are completed with a detailed examination of the contractile tissue function of all the muscles attaching to the lumbo-pelvic-hip complex. The presence and the location of pain evoked during resisted testing is correlated with the muscle's strength, thus enabling the therapist to reach a diagnosis of muscle 'sprain' and/or rupture. Grades 1 and 2 muscle sprains are painfully strong when resisted isometrically as opposed to Grade 3 sprains (i.e. complete ruptures) which are relatively painfree and weak when resisted isometrically. Of course, there exists an entire spectrum of dysfunction

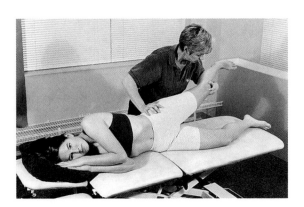

Figure 7.60   Test for extensibility of the middle band of tensor fascia lata (Kendall et al 1993).

between the two extremes. It must be remembered that contractions of muscles induce compression forces across joints and also increase tension in the various ligaments to which they attach. Therefore, a pain response may not be indicative of a muscle strain at all, but rather the pain may be coming from a joint which reacts to compression or from a ligament which is painful to stretch.

Neurological tests

These tests examine the conductivity of the motor and sensory nerves relative to the lumbosacral plexus as well as the mobility of the dura through the intervertebral foramina.

Motor tests

The L2 to S2 motor nerve roots are evaluated clinically via the peripheral muscles they innervate. Although there are no true peripheral myotomes in the lower quadrant (one muscle solely innervated by one nerve root), specific muscles known as *key muscles* are primarily innervated by one motor nerve and their function is a reflection of the neurological innervation. Initially, a maximal contraction is elicited from the key muscle and the quantity and quality of strength are compared to the opposite side. If the muscle tests are strong, six submaximal contractions are elicited to detect accelerated fatiguability—a common finding of neurological impedance.

The motor nerves and the key muscles which are evaluated include:

L2 — iliopsoas, adductors
L3 — adductors, quadriceps
L4 — quadriceps, tibialus anterior
L5 — extensor hallucis, extensor digitorum, peronei
S1 — hamstrings, gastrocnemius
S2 — hamstrings, gluteus maximus.

Sensory tests

The L1 to S2 sensory nerve roots are evaluated

clinically via the dermatomes they innervate. Dermatome maps can be confusing since variations in dermatome distribution exist from individual to individual. Furthermore, impedance of sensory conductivity may be reflected in a range of dysaesthesia from slight hyperaesthesia to complete anaesthesia. Detailed examination of the distal extent of the dermatome is useful in detecting early neurological interference. One of the first signs of sensory dysfunction is hyperaesthesia within a specific dermatome. This sign tends to occur long before sensation becomes reduced or obliterated completely and its existence is often a surprise to the patient.

Although individual variability is recognized, the following description of dermatome distribution is one commonly seen:

L1 — upper posterior buttock, anterior groin
L2 — middle posterior buttock, anterior thigh to the knee
L3 — lower posterior buttock, anterior thigh to the medial knee and occasionally distal to the medial malleolus
L4 — lateral thigh, medial leg, dorsum of the foot to the great toe
L5 — lateral leg, dorsum of the foot to toes 2, 3, 4, sole of the foot (excluding the heel) to toes 1, 2, 3
S1 — posterior thigh, leg, lateral border of the foot to dorsum and sole, to toes 4 and 5
S2 — posterior thigh, leg to heel
S3, S4 — perineal region.

Reflex tests

The spinal reflexes are evaluated via the myotatic response to stretch of the key muscle innervated by the root in question. They include the following:

L3, L4 — quadriceps (i.e. knee jerk)
L5, S1, S2 — gastrocnemius (i.e. ankle jerk).

The integrity of the spinal cord is evaluated by the plantar response test.

Dural mobility tests

The mobility of the dura mater surrounding the L2 to S2 nerve roots is evaluated by two tests, the femoral nerve stretch test and the straight leg raise test.

Femoral nerve stretch test. With the patient prone, the lower extremity is palpated above the ankle. The lower leg is passively flexed at the knee joint and the quantity and end feel of motion are noted. When the mobility of the dura mater of the L2, L3 and/or L4 nerve roots is restricted, hip extension and knee flexion are restricted by pain felt posteriorly in the lumbar spine.

Straight leg raise test. With the patient lying supine, the lower extremity is palpated above the ankle. While maintaining the knee in extension and the femur in slight adduction/medial rotation, the femur is flexed at the hip joint. The quantity and end feel of motion are noted. When the mobility of the dura mater of the L4, L5, S1, and/or S2 nerve roots is restricted, hip flexion is limited to 30° to 60° by both pain and muscle spasm.

Vascular tests

These tests screen the circulatory status of the lower extremity. Careful observation of the skin color, texture, response to dependency and elevation and the length of time for superficial wounds to heal should be noted. The femoral, popliteal and dorsalis pedis arteries are palpated and auscultated in the femoral triangle, popliteal fossa and dorsum of the foot respectively. If a deep vein thrombophlebitis is suspected, the response to passive dorsiflexion of the ankle should be noted (Homans' sign) and the region carefully palpated for heat and/or tenderness.

Adjunctive tests

X-rays make good policemen but poor counselors, in that while the straight radiography may exclude serious bone disease and significant mechanical defect, it does not often provide much guidance about how to treat the patient (Grieve 1981).

The primary reason for obtaining the results of adjunctive tests is to rule out serious pathology and to discover the presence of anatomical anomalies prior to treatment.

The adjunctive tests available include the following:

1. radiography (X-rays)
2. discography
3. myelography
4. radiculography
5. epidurography
6. tomography
7. transverse axial tomography
8. computed transverse axial tomography
9. radiographic stereoplotting
10. interosseous spinal venography
11. cineradiography and fluoroscopy
12. thermography
13. nerve root infiltration
14. electrodiagnosis
15. intervertebral disc manometry
16. cystometry
17. radioactive isotope studies
18. ultrasonography
19. nuclear magnetic resonance.

With respect to the sacroiliac joint, Lawson et al (1982) reported on the benefits of computed axial tomography (CT scanning techniques) as opposed to conventional radiography in the detection of mild erosions and narrowing of the joint. Because of the three-dimensional spatial orientation of the sacroiliac joint, CT scanning was superior in obtaining visualization of the joint space. Thus the diagnosis of inflammatory sacroiliitis, which is based on the identification of joint narrowing, sclerosis, ankylosis or erosion, was facilitated. Figures 7.62 to 7.65 illustrate the visualization of both the synovial and the ligamentous portions of the sacroiliac joint that is possible with this adjunctive test.

CT scanning techniques can reveal congenital and/or acquired anatomical changes at the lumbosacral junction (Fig. 7.66). The dimensions of the central spinal canal as well as the lateral recess are clearly visualized and often confirm or negate the clinical findings of physical trespass.

The lumbosacral junction is often the site of congenital anomalies which may or may not be significant to the clinical picture. Their presence,

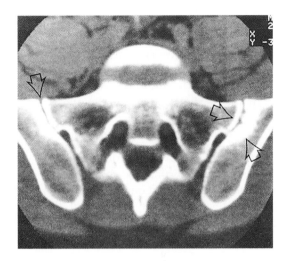

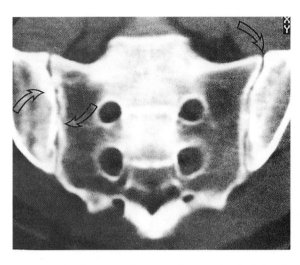

Figure 7.62 A computed tomography scan (transverse plane) of a patient with Reiter's disease. This technique clearly reveals the focal sclerosis (arrows), narrowing and erosion of the sacroiliac joint associated with this disease. The depth of the joint is clearly visualized.

Figure 7.63 A computed tomography scan (vertical plane) of a patient with Reiter's disease illustrating narrowing, erosion and focal sclerosis (arrows) of the articular surfaces of the sacroiliac joints.

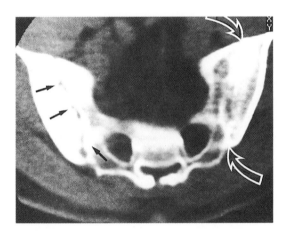

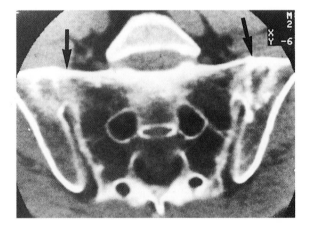

Figure 7.64 A computed tomography scan of a patient with ankylosing spondylitis. Note the total ankylosis of the right sacroiliac joint (open arrows).

Figure 7.65 A computed tomography scan of a patient with ankylosing spondylitis. Note the bilateral bony ankylosis of the sacroiliac joints. (Figs 7.62–7.65 are reproduced from Lawson et al 1982 with permission of the publishers Raven Press.)

however, should be ascertained. The anomalies which are seen at this level include:

1. asymmetry of the posterior zygapophyseal joints
2. congenital absence of a pedicle
3. accessory laminae
4. osseous bridging of the transverse processes

5. dysplasia or absence of the spinous process of the L5 or S1 vertebrae (spina bifida)
6. dysplasia of the pars interarticularis
7. spina magna of the L5 vertebra
8. trapezoidal L5 vertebra, lumbarized S1 vertebra; partial or complete

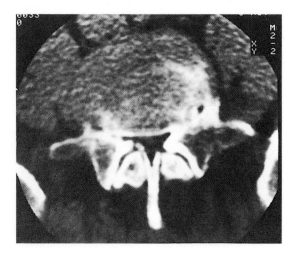

Figure 7.66   A computed tomography scan of the L5–S1 segment, illustrating central stenosis secondary to enlargement of the zygapophyseal joints bilaterally. (Reproduced with permission from Kirkaldy-Willis 1983.)

9. sacralized L5 vertebra; partial or complete
10. anomalous adventitious joint between the transverse process of the L5 vertebra and the ala of the sacrum
11. asymmetric height of the ala of the sacrum with one side higher than the other creating a 'sacral tilt'
12. calcified iliolumbar ligament (Grieve 1981).

The findings noted on adjunctive testing of the lumbo-pelvic-hip complex must be correlated with the findings noted on clinical examination if their significance is to be understood. Rarely can treatment be directed by the results of these tests alone.

8

Lumbosacral junction: clinical syndromes

CLASSIFICATION

Lumbosacral disorders have been classified (MacNab 1977) as visceral, vascular, neurogenic, psychogenic, sociogenic and/or spondylogenic in origin. Briefly, disorders of the pelvic viscera can refer pain to the lumbar region and are easily confused with benign mechanical dysfunction. Insufficiency of the peripheral vascular system can secondarily give rise to backache and/or symptoms resembling sciatica. Neurogenic disorders include benign and/or malignant tumours of the central or peripheral nervous system. A central lesion at the lumbosacral junction can mimic a cauda equina compression lesion. Pure psychogenic or sociogenic backache is not often seen although stress can play a role in magnifying the perception of pain.

Spondylogenic disorders have been further classified (MacNab 1977) as:

1. Pathologic soft tissue and bony
  a. Scheuermann's disease—vertebral
    osteochondritis
  b. Infective—pyogenic vertebral
    osteomyelitis
  c. Systemic inflammatory—rheumatoid
    arthritis, ankylosing spondylitis
  d. Metabolic—osteoporosis, Paget's disease,
    tuberculosis, Calvé's disease, DISH
    (diffuse idiopathic skeletal hyperostosis)
2. Traumatic soft tissue and bony
  a. Fractures
  b. Contusions
  c. Spondylolisthesis/spondylolysis

3. Aging, adaptation, degeneration
   a. Arthrosis of the posterior zygapophyseal joints
   b. Spondylosis of the intervertebral disc.

Systemic and/or inflammatory disorders affecting the lumbosacral region can be differentiated clinically from traumatic inflammation (i.e. sprain) by the lack of trauma in the history, the inconsistent response of the joint to both mechanical stress and to rest, as well as the lack of resolution with appropriate therapy over a short period of time. The experienced clinician will quickly recognize the pattern of response to therapy which deviates from the norm, and will question the biomechanical pathogenesis at this point. Subsequent investigation is then indicated.

Although scientific verification of the anatomical and physiological factors responsible for nociception is essential for specific diagnosis, prognosis and classifications such as those above, this rarely enhances our ability to treat the patient. For the clinician, classifications which follow a biomechanical model based on mobility and stability have proven more useful and provide a consistent therapeutic approach. In keeping with this model, lumbosacral disorders can be classified into three groups, each of which describes the objective findings noted on mobility testing and suggests the appropriate restorative therapy. They include:

1. hypomobility with or without pain
2. hypermobility/instability with or without pain
3. normal mobility with pain.

This classification pertains to the osteokinematic function of lumbosacral junction which depends on the arthrokinematic and myokinematic function of L5–S1 (see Ch. 5). This classification does not provide a specific anatomical nor physiological cause for the aberrant mobility noted; however, since mobilization and stabilization techniques used in manual therapy are specific to restoring movement patterns, the cause is not always required for formulating treatment plans. The aim of all evaluation procedures is to identify the system (i.e. articular vs. myofascial) which is aberrantly altering the osteokinematic function of the L5 vertebra during functional movement. Subsequently, treatment can be directed to the articular and/or myofascial system. If the biomechanics of the lumbo-pelvic-hip region are restored in accordance with those presented in Chapter 5, symptomatic and objective improvement usually follows, but only if the underlying etiology is biomechanical in nature.

HYPOMOBILITY WITH OR WITHOUT PAIN

The physiological and anatomical changes which accompany lumbosacral dysfunction in this category have been described and beautifully illustrated by Kirkaldy-Willis & Hill (1979), Kirkaldy-Willis (1983) and Taylor & Twomey (1986, 1992). The essential objective finding for classification here is *decreased* osteokinematic motion of the L5 vertebra relative to the sacrum. The etiology of restriction may be either articular, myofascial or both and is commonly the result of an excessive rotational or compressive force which exceeded the physiological range of the unit (Bogduk 1997, Farfan 1973, Gracovetsky & Farfan 1986, Gracovetsky et al 1981, Kirkaldy-Willis et al 1978, Kirkaldy-Willis 1983, Taylor et al 1990, Twomey et al 1989).

The specific anatomical and physiological changes include:

1. synovitis of the posterior zygapophyseal joints (Grade 1–2 sprain), strain of the iliolumbar ligament
2. minor circumferential tears of the outer layers of the annulus and the associated anterior and posterior longitudinal ligaments (Fig. 8.1)
3. minor joint subluxations
4. end-plate fractures (compression overload, rarely seen at the lumbosacral junction) (Bogduk 1997, Farfan 1978, Kirkaldy-Willis 1983)
5. hypertonic segmental posterior musculature
6. in more severe injuries, tears of the capsule and ligamentum flavum as well as

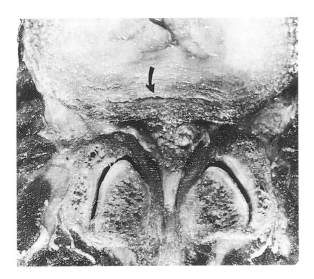

Figure 8.1   A transverse circumferential tear in the annulus fibrosis (arrow). (Reproduced with permission from Kirkaldy-Willis 1983.)

subchondral fractures of the superior articular process have been noted (Taylor et al 1990). These injuries were not evident on X-ray.

Subjective findings

The mode of onset may be either insidious or sudden, and depends on the degree of trauma encountered. The presence or absence of pain depends on mechanical and/or chemical irritation of the local nociceptors which in turn is a function of the stage of the pathology (substrate, fibroblastic, maturation). The pain may be unilateral or bilateral and is usually localized to the lumbosacral junction with occasional radiation to the buttock. Dysaesthesia is not often reported. The aggravating activities include the extremes of range of motion of forward/backward bending, prolonged standing and lifting. Rest usually affords relief.

Objective findings

Mobility

In the first few days after injury (substrate phase), the patient with acute symptoms

presents with marked restriction in all ranges of motion. Both forward and backward bending are limited as well as lateral bending to the left and right. The range of motion is bilaterally limited when the pathology is bilateral, and unilaterally limited when the pathology is unilateral. There may be a localized kyphosis and/or rotation evident at the lumbosacral junction (Fig. 8.2) secondary to the hypertonic lumbar longissimus muscle whose orientation (see Ch. 4) retracts the L5 vertebra (Bogduk 1997). The severity of the pain usually restricts a detailed mobility assessment at this stage; however, with resolution over the next few days, mobility testing (see Ch. 7) confirms the restricted osteokinematic function of the L5–S1 segment.

During the fibroblastic stage, unilateral restrictions of flexion and/or extension may produce a multisegmental rotoscoliosis during

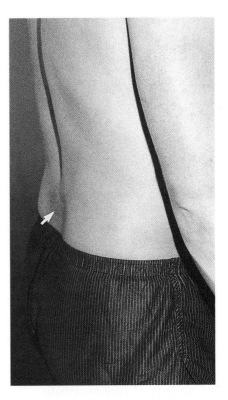

Figure 8.2   Localized rotation of the L5 vertebra (arrow) secondary to hypertonicity of the lumbar longissimus muscle.

forward and/or backward bending of the trunk, manifested both during the osteokinematic and positional testing of the lumbar spine. This is the first sign that an underlying restriction exists, since neither rotation nor sideflexion should occur coupled with flexion/extension during forward or backward bending of the trunk (in the presence of a level sacral base; see Ch. 5). The ipsilateral posterior rotation test (Gillet) may also be adversely affected by the hypomobile lesion.

In the initial stages of injury, arthrokinematic testing specific to the L5–S1 segment reveals a full range of articular motion. Palpation of the hypertonic segmental musculature confirms the myofascial etiology of the restriction. Treatment should be directed towards restoring the function of the myofascial system (active mobilization techniques).

If restrictive capsular adhesions develop, the arthrokinematic function will be reduced and the joint restriction confirmed on testing. Treatment should now be directed towards both the articular system (passive mobilization techniques) as well as the myofascial system (active mobilization techniques) for full restoration of function.

Stability

Lumbosacral disorders in this category do not exhibit a loss of arthrokinetic function. After the initial acute stage has subsided, the passive stability tests are tested and are normal. Muscle control, however, has been shown to be adversely affected (Hides et al 1994, 1996) in acute low back injuries and the force closure system (inner unit control) will be affected.

Neurological tests

All tests for neurological conductivity and neural mobility relative to the lumbosacral junction are normal.

Classification of hypomobile dysfunction

The segmental restriction can be subclassified

according to the position in which the L5 vertebra is held. A Flexed L5 vertebra exhibits a bilateral restriction of extension, whereas an Extended L5 vertebra exhibits a bilateral restriction of flexion. The unilateral lesions produce a segmental rotation of the L5 vertebra as well as a compensatory multisegmental curve above the L5 vertebra. A Flexed Rotated/Sideflexed Left (FRSL) L5 vertebra exhibits a restriction of extension and right rotation/sideflexion, whereas an Extended Rotated/Sideflexed Left (ERSL) L5 vertebra exhibits a restriction of flexion and right rotation/sideflexion. Note that this terminology does not identify the pathogenesis of the restriction.

Treatment of the hypomobile lumbosacral junction

Treatment of the lumbosacral junction forms part of the overall rehabilitation of the lumbo-pelvic-hip complex. The ultimate goal is to restore the biomechanics of the entire region, part of which requires the optimal function of L5–S1. The following section outlines the specific therapy indicated during each stage of repair (i.e. substrate, fibroblastic, maturation) when localized hypomobility of L5–S1 is found.

The myofascial component of therapy (restoration of the force closure mechanism) pertinent to the lumbo-pelvic-hip region will be discussed in Chapter 11.

Substrate phase

During the first 4 to 6 days after injury, the goal of treatment is hemostasis of the wound. At home, the frequent application of ice together with rest is the treatment of choice. The resting position of the lumbar spine (Fig. 8.3) is the supine position with the hips and knees semiflexed and supported over a wedge. The surface should be firm, but not rigid.

At the clinic, electrotherapeutic analgesic modalities such as transcutaneous nerve stimulation and interferential current therapy can afford relief from pain; however, the patient

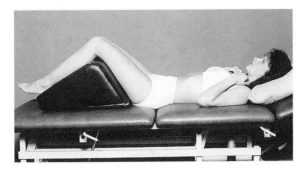

Figure 8.3   The resting position of the lumbar spine.

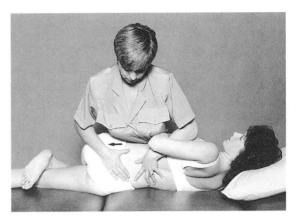

Figure 8.4   Passive mobilization: specific traction of the lumbosacral junction. The arrow indicates the direction of force applied to the patient's pelvic girdle.

should not attend at this stage if the physical stresses induced are greater than the relief gained.

Fibroblastic phase

With the resolution of active range of movement, the specific osteokinematic restriction becomes apparent. During this stage of repair, the goal of treatment is twofold, that is, to restore the segmental articular mobility (kinematics) as well as the tensile strength of the unit (kinetics). Passive and active mobilization techniques are used to restore the articular kinematics, and combined with ultrasound and laser for the enhancement of collagen production (tensile strength) at the wound site (Abergel 1984, Bassett 1968, Mester 1971, Webster et al 1980). In addition, a specific home exercise program designed to maintain and increase articular mobility is given. Details of the treatment for two hypomobile lumbosacral dysfunctions in this stage of repair are outlined below.

Flexed rotated/sideflexed left (FRSL) L5–S1

Specific traction: passive mobilization technique (Fig. 8.4). This is a useful preliminary mobilization technique which can be graded according to the irritability of the joint. Initially, gentle grades are indicated, keeping well within the range of pain and reactive muscle spasm. The large afferent fiber input from the large mechanoreceptors located in the articular capsule inhibits the centripetal transmission of

the small fiber input (nociception) at the spinal cord, thus reducing the perception of pain via the spinal gating mechanism (see Ch. 4).

The stimulation of these mechanoreceptors also reduces the gamma efferent discharge to the intrafusal muscle fiber of the segmentally related muscle, thus reducing hypertonicity. If the myofascia is primarily responsible for the restriction of osteokinematic function, this technique should certainly be included in the early treatment plan.

With the patient sidelying, hips and knees slightly flexed, the interspinous space between the L4 and the L5 vertebra is palpated with the caudal hand. The thoracolumbar spine is rotated by pulling the patient's lower arm forward until rotation of L4–L5 occurs. The cranial hand now palpates the interspinous space between the L5 vertebra and the sacrum while the caudal hand flexes the patient's uppermost hip and knee. Simultaneously, the patient should extend the lower leg to the end of the table. The foot of the upper leg is allowed to rest against the popliteal fossa of the lower leg. The therapist's lower lateral thorax contacts the patient's uppermost innominate.

Specific traction is applied to the lumbosacral junction via a straight caudal force from the therapist's lower lateral thorax against the patient's pelvic girdle. The therapist's cranial arm stabilizes the patient's upper thorax. The degree of force applied is dictated by the joint/myofascial reaction.

Rotation/sideflexion: passive and active mobilization techniques. The rotation/sideflexion component of the osteokinematic restriction is usually myofascial in origin at this stage of repair since restrictive capsular adhesions have not had time to form. Grades 2 and 3 (Grieve 1981) rotation/sideflexion passive mobilization techniques are utilized for their neurophysiological effect on the segmental myofascia, that is the reduction in hypertonicity and subsequently the return of osteokinematic function. The technique yields the best result when it is used in combination with the active mobilization technique (see below).

Localization. With the patient in left sidelying, hips and knees slightly flexed, the interspinous space between the L4 and the L5 vertebra is palpated with the caudal hand. The thoracolumbar spine is rotated by pulling the patient's lower arm forward until rotation of L4–L5 occurs. Comfort is assured if techniques are focused and localized and full articular locking is avoided (Hartman 1997). The cranial hand now palpates the interspinous space between the L5 vertebra and the sacrum while the caudal hand flexes the patient's uppermost hip and knee. Simultaneously, the patient should extend the lower leg to the end of the table. The foot of the upper leg is allowed to rest against the popliteal fossa of the lower leg. The therapist's cranial arm supports the patient's thorax while the caudal arm supports the pelvic girdle.

Passive mobilization (Fig. 8.5). From the above position, L5–S1 is passively mobilized into extension and right rotation/sideflexion through either the thorax or the pelvic girdle. The technique is graded according to the joint/myofascial reaction.

Active mobilization (Fig. 8.6). L5–S1 is initially mobilized passively into extension and right rotation/sideflexion. From the point of first resistance, the patient is instructed to resist further motion while the therapist applies a gentle rotation force to the pelvic girdle or the thorax. The isometric contraction is held for up

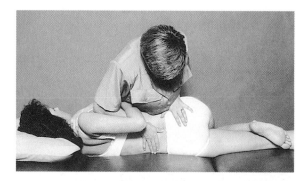

Figure 8.5 Passive mobilization for extension and right rotation/sideflexion of the lumbosacral junction.

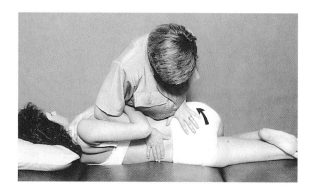

Figure 8.6 Active mobilization for extension and right rotation/sideflexion of the lumbosacral junction. The arrow indicates the direction of resistance applied by the therapist.

to 5 seconds followed by a period of complete relaxation. The joint is then passively taken to the new physiological range of extension and right rotation/sideflexion. The technique is repeated three times followed by re-evaluation of osteokinematic function. These techniques should be dynamic, since holding a joint at the limit of its physiological range can be irritating and provoke a reactive muscle spasm response.

Home exercise program. A home exercise program designed to restore segmental osteokinematic function at the lumbosacral junction is paramount to successful rehabilitation. Since wound repair occurs throughout 24 hours, the orientation of the newly formed collagen fibers should be directed as often as possible (see Ch. 6).

In the early fibroblastic stage of repair, gentle range of motion exercises well within the

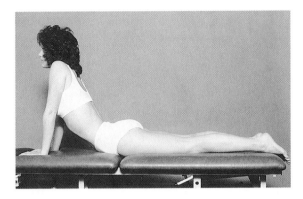

Figure 8.7 Passive press-ups, the initial exercise given for mobilization of the flexed rotated/sideflexed left (FRSL) lesion, should be repeated frequently.

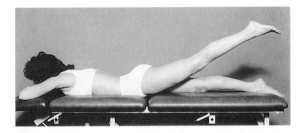

Figure 8.8 Unilateral left leg raises for mobilization of the FRSL lesion.

painfree range are indicated. The hypomobile lumbosacral junction which is held in the flexed, left rotated/sideflexed (FRSL) position requires an exercise program aimed at restoring extension and right rotation/sideflexion. Passive press-ups (Fig. 8.7) from the prone position repeated frequently are the initial exercises given. Subsequently, unilateral left leg raises from the prone position (Fig. 8.8) producing intra-pelvic torsion and right lumbosacral rotation (see Ch. 5), can be added.

Extended rotated/sideflexed right (ERSR) L5–S1

Specific traction: passive mobilization technique (Fig. 8.4). As with the FRSL lesion, specific traction is a useful preliminary mobilization technique which can be graded according to the irritability of the joint. The

details and the intent of this technique are identical to those described above.

Rotation/sideflexion: passive and active mobilization techniques. See the section on the FRSL lesion for details on the intent of these techniques during the fibroblastic stage of repair.

Localization. With the patient in right side-lying, hips and knees slightly flexed, the interspinous space between the L4 and the L5 vertebra is palpated with the caudal hand. The thoracolumbar spine is rotated by pulling the patient's lower arm until rotation of L4–L5 occurs. Comfort is assured if techniques are focused and localized and full articular locking is avoided (Hartman 1997). The cranial hand now palpates the interspinous space between the L5 vertebra and the sacrum while the caudal hand flexes the patient's uppermost hip and knee. Simultaneously, the patient should extend the lower leg to the end of the table. The foot of the upper leg is allowed to rest against the popliteal fossa of the lower leg. The therapist's cranial arm supports the patient's thorax while the caudal arm supports the pelvic girdle.

Passive mobilization (Fig. 8.9). From the above position, L5–S1 is passively mobilized into flexion and left rotation/sideflexion through either the thorax or the pelvic girdle. The technique is graded according to the joint/myofascial reaction.

Active mobilization (Fig. 8.10). L5–S1 is initially mobilized passively into flexion and left

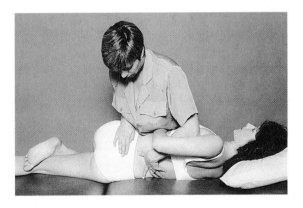

Figure 8.9 Passive mobilization for flexion and left rotation/sideflexion of the lumbosacral junction.

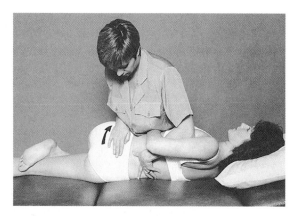

Figure 8.10 Active mobilization for flexion and left rotation/sideflexion of the lumbosacral junction. The arrow indicates the direction of resistance applied by the therapist.

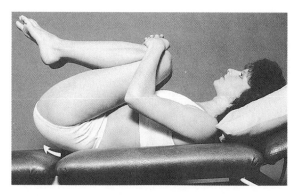

Figure 8.11 Passive curl-ups, the initial exercise for mobilization of the extended rotated sideflexed right (ERSR) lesion, should be repeated frequently.

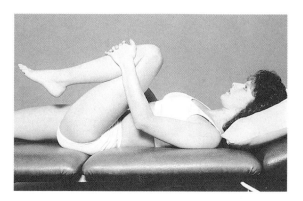

Figure 8.12 Unilateral flexion of the left hip in the supine position for mobilization of the ERSR lesion.

rotation/sideflexion. From the point of first resistance, the patient is instructed to resist further motion while the therapist applies a gentle rotation force to the pelvic girdle or the thorax. The isometric contraction is held for up to 5 seconds followed by a period of complete relaxation. The joint is then passively taken to the new physiological range of flexion and left rotation/sideflexion. The technique is repeated three times followed by re-evaluation of osteokinematic function. These techniques should be dynamic, since holding a joint at the limit of its physiological range can be irritating and provoke a reactive muscle spasm response.

Home exercise program. A home exercise program designed to restore segmental osteokinematic function at the lumbosacral junction is paramount to successful rehabilitation. Since wound repair occurs throughout 24 h, the orientation of the newly formed collagen fibers should be directed as often as possible (see Ch. 6).

In the early fibroblastic stage of repair, gentle range of motion exercises, well within the painfree range, are indicated. The hypomobile lumbosacral junction which is held in the extended, right rotated/sideflexed (ERSR) position requires an exercise program aimed at restoring flexion and left rotation/sideflexion. Passive curl-ups (Fig. 8.11) from the supine position repeated frequently are the initial exercises given. Subsequently, unilateral flexion of the left hip (Fig. 8.12) in the supine position

producing intra-pelvic torsion and left lumbosacral rotation (see Ch. 5), can be added.

Maturation phase

If restrictive capsular adhesions have developed during the fibroblastic stage of repair, stronger passive mobilization techniques will be required to restore the optimal kinematic function of the lumbosacral junction. In addition, a vigorous home exercise program designed to reorganize the collagen fibers within the adhesion will be necessary.

The active and passive mobilization techniques utilized at this stage of repair are identical to those previously described except that the joint is taken strongly and specifically to the limit

---

Box 8.1 Case history

A 27-year-old warehouse worker presented at the clinic 2 days after the onset of low back pain following a heavy day of repetitive lifting and twisting. During one such lift, he noted an acute twinge of pain in his low back which forced him to remain in a kyphotic position for several minutes. Eventually he was able to straighten up and immediately reported for first aid. Subsequent to seeing his family physician, he was referred to physiotherapy for evaluation and treatment.

This was the first episode of low back pain which had forced his absence from work. He had experienced low back pain in the past from which he had been able to recover spontaneously with rest. The pain was located at the lumbosacral junction with bilateral radiation into both buttocks. Dysaesthesia was not reported. The aggravating factors included all extremes of motion, in particular, forward bending.

Initially, objective examination was limited by the severity of the pain evoked on movement testing. Osteokinematically, all motions of the lumbo-pelvic-hip complex were restricted. Over the next few days, as the acute inflammatory stage (substrate phase) subsided, the functional tests revealed an asymmetry of motion of the L5 vertebra relative to the sacrum on forward bending, such that the right transverse process travelled further superiorly than the left. Subsequent articular mobility tests exposed a segmental restriction of flexion and right rotation/sideflexion of L5–S1. The arthrokinetic

and neurological tests were normal. The segmental musculature was hypertonic to palpation and reactive to stretch, suggesting a myofascial etiology. This lesion can be classified as an ERSL: the joint is held in a position of extension and rotation/sideflexion to the left and limited in flexion and rotation/sideflexion to the right.

The patient was advised to rest in the supine position with a wedge or support beneath the semi-flexed knees and to apply ice to the lumbar spine frequently. On the 6th day after injury, gentle passive and active mobilization was begun. The techniques chosen included specific traction, passive flexion and right rotation/sideflexion combined with an active mobilization in the same direction. Interferential current therapy was given as an electrotherapeutic analgesic and the patient was sent home with gentle flexion exercises (curl-ups) to be kept well within the painfree range.

The patient was seen three times weekly over the next 3 weeks during which the lumbosacral junction was progressively mobilized until optimal osteokinematic function had returned. At least 6 months of healing time is required before the tensile strength of the damaged tissue is restored; therefore, careful review of proper ergonomics (see Ch. 11) was a crucial part of this patient's rehabilitation. In addition, attention was given to the function of the inner unit of muscles (multifidus and transversus abdominis) so that recurrence could be avoided (Hides et al 1994, 1996) (see Ch. 11).

---

of the physiological range of motion (Grade 4). Grade 5 (high velocity, low amplitude thrust) techniques are indicated when the joint irritability is low and the end feel of motion is very hard. The localization and positioning for the Grade 5 technique is identical to that previously described. The direction of the thrust is critical to the success of the technique and must be about the appropriate oblique axis of rotation.

The specific exercises given in the maturation stage of repair are identical to those described above, with the exception that they need not be contained within the painfree range of motion; however, the quality of the pain induced as well as its duration should be minimal. Exercises for global lumbo-pelvic-hip function (see Ch. 11) should also be included.

HYPERMOBILITY/INSTABILITY WITH OR WITHOUT PAIN

Repeated trauma to the lumbosacral junction can

result in progressive anatomical and physiological changes leading to segmental instability (Table 8.1) (Bogduk 1997, Kirkaldy-Willis 1983, Panjabi 1992). The essential objective finding for classification here is the presence of *increased* osteokinematic motion of the L5 vertebra relative to the sacrum (increased neutral zone). When the angular motion of the segment is increased but the linear translation is within normal limits with a good solid end feel, the joint is classified as hypermobile. When both the angular and linear motion is increased, the joint is classified as unstable. When a joint is unstable, the linear motion often occurs in the opposite direction from normal. For example, flexion is normally coupled with anterior translation. When the segment is unstable, it is not uncommon to see flexion coupled with posterior translation and extension coupled with anterior translation.

Following extreme or repeated rotational and/or posteroanterior shear trauma, the following anatomical and physiological changes can occur.

Table 8.1 The degenerative process (from Kirkaldy-Willis 1983)

ZYGAPOPHYSEAL JOINTS		INTERVERTEBRAL DISC
Synovitis ↓	DYSFUNCTION	Circumferential tears ↓
Fibrillation of articular cartilage ↓		Radial tears (herniation) ↓
Capsular laxity and continued cartilage destruction ↓	INSTABILITY	Internal disruption ↓ ↓
Subluxation → ↓	Lateral nerve entrapment	← Disc resorption ↓
Enlargement of articular process →	STABILIZATION One level stenosis ↓	← Osteophytosis
	Multilevel spondylosis and stenosis occurs as a result of recurrent strains	

1. Fibrillation and subsequent loss of the articular cartilage of the zygapophyseal joint(s) (Figs 8.13, 8.14) (Bogduk 1997, Taylor & Twomey 1986).
2. Laxity of the articular capsule(s) and attenuation of the iliolumbar ligament.
3. Fracture of the articular process with resultant strain deformation of the neural arch (Taylor et al 1990, Twomey et al 1989).
4. Coalescence of the circumferential annular tears into a radial fissure (Fig. 8.15) with/without subsequent herniation of the nucleus pulposus, ultimately progressing to marked internal disruption of the disc, loss of disc height, circumferential bulging and resorption.

5. Sclerosis of the adjacent vertebral bodies (Fig. 8.16).

At the lumbosacral junction, these anatomical changes allow the superior articular process of the sacrum to sublux upwards and forwards during axial rotation of the trunk (Fig. 8.17). This motion consequently narrows the lateral recess of L5–S1, potentially impeding the vascular and neurological function of the structures within the intervertebral foramen (Sunderland 1978).

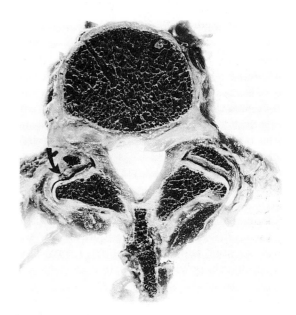

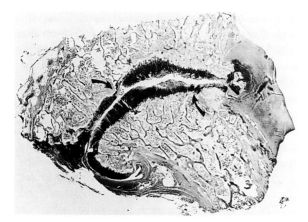

Figure 8.13 Histological section of the zygapophyseal joint. Note the thinning and fibrillation of the articular cartilage (arrows).

Figure 8.14 Macroscopic transverse section of the L5–S1 segment. Note the marked degeneration of the left zygapophyseal joint (arrow).

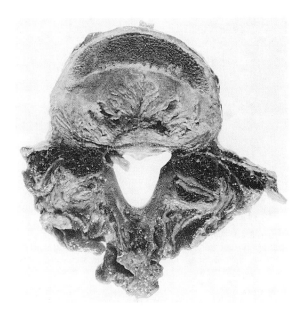

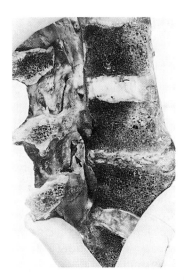

Figure 8.15 Macroscopic transverse section of the L4–L5 segment. Note the coalescence of several radial fissures and the early stages of internal disruption. (Figs 8.13–8.15 reproduced with permission from Kirkaldy-Willis 1983.)

Figure 8.17 Dynamic stenosis of the lateral recess of the lumbosacral junction associated with instability. In this specimen the spinous process of the L5 vertebra has been rotated towards the observer. The zygapophyseal joint has opened (arrow), the superior articular process has approximated the posterior aspect of the intervertebral disc subsequently narrowing the lateral recess. (Reproduced with permission from Reilly J et al 1978.)

Subjective findings

Clinically, the patient with a hypermobile/unstable lumbosacral junction presents with a long history of intermittent low back pain with repeat episodes of exacerbation and resolution. The presence or absence of pain depends on mechanical and/or chemical irritation of the local nociceptors, as well as the individual's overall level of mobility. The pain may be unilateral or bilateral and can be referred as far as the distal extent of the L5 or S1 dermatome. Dysaesthesia is common given the potential for neurovascular impedance at the intervertebral foramen. The aggravating activities depend on which anatomical structure is currently responsible for nociceptive transmission. Disorders of the neural arch frequently resemble the hypomobile lesion subjectively, in that extreme ranges of motion, lifting and prolonged standing can be aggravating activities. When the intervertebral disc is responsible for pain production, compressive activities such as prolonged sitting and flexion are intolerable. Rest usually affords relief.

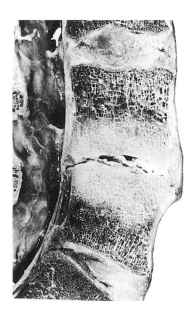

Figure 8.16 Macroscopic sagittal section of the lumbar spine. Note the sclerosis of the vertebral bodies above and below the central intervertebral disc which is markedly resorbed. (Reproduced with permission from Kirkaldy-Willis et al 1978.)

Objective findings

Mobility

Objectively, the hypermobile/unstable patient may adopt altered lumbo-pelvic-hip movement patterns to compensate for the loss of ability to transfer load through the lumbosacral junction. Typically, they forward bend by walking their hands down their thighs and back up to return to erect standing (Fig. 8.18). Alternatively, they may forward or backward bend by flexing or extending the pelvic girdle on the hip joints without involving the spinal segments at all. Often, a deep skin crease is noted at the unstable level during backward bending of the trunk (Fig. 8.19). The normal lumbo-pelvic-hip rhythm during functional movement may even be reversed (see Ch. 5).

Specific mobility testing of the lumbosacral junction reveals increased mobility of flexion/extension and/or sideflexion/rotation. The presence or absence of pain on these tests depends on the level of irritability of the joint at the time of evaluation. Commonly, a patient with acute low back pain will initially present with a hypomobile segment due to the reactive muscle

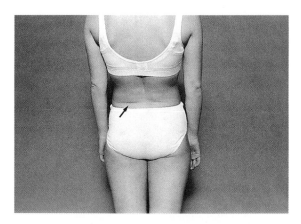

Figure 8.19 When segmental hypermobility of posteroanterior translation is present, backward bending of the trunk will produce a localized deep skin crease (arrow).

spasm. With resolution, the underlying hypermobile/unstable joint is revealed.

Stability

The arthrokinetic tests for shear and torsion are always positive for pain and excess range of motion when the segment is unstable. The inner unit of muscles is reflexively inhibited and Hodges & Richardson (1996) have shown that there is a timing delay in the recruitment of these muscles during functional tasks when instability is present.

Neurological tests

Impedance of neurological function (motor, sensory, reflex) and neural mobility is common in patients with instability but not hypermobility. Instability can interfere with the dimensions of the lateral recess during rotation. This potentially impedes the neurovascular bundle (Figs 8.20, 8.21) and at the lumbosacral junction, the L5 nerve root would be affected. Centrally, the annulus can protrude or herniate, thus reducing the dimensions of the spinal canal and consequently interfering with the S1 nerve root. In both instances, the slump and the straight leg raise test for neural mobility would be adversely affected.

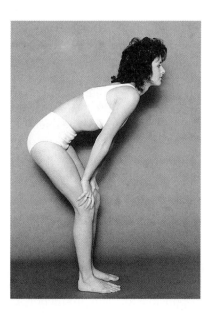

Figure 8.18 Typical pattern of forward bending of the trunk when stability is lost at the lumbosacral junction.

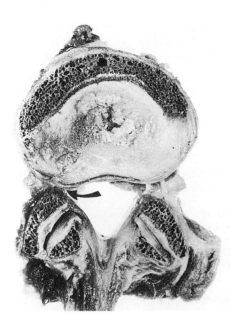

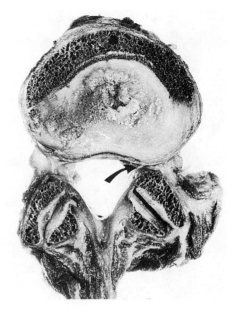

Figure 8.20   Macroscopic transverse section of the L4–L5 segment demonstrating the effect of instability on the dimensions of the lateral recess. Note the approximation of the superior articular process towards the intervertebral disc on the left during axial rotation and the subsequent obliteration of the left lateral recess (arrow). (Reproduced with permission from Kirkaldy-Willis 1983.)

Figure 8.21   The same specimen as in Figure 8.20 axially rotated in the opposite direction. Note the approximation of the superior articular process towards the intervertebral disc on the right (compare with Figure 8.20) and the subsequent obliteration of the right lateral recess (arrow). (Reproduced with permission from Kirkaldy-Willis 1983.)

The spectrum of neurological impedance is variable and depends on the degree of pathology. The patient may present with minimal motor weakness or sensory dysaesthesia in the early stages, and later with a complete motor nerve block and sensory anaesthesia. Careful objective evaluation is mandatory to detect the early neurological decompensation.

End results

With time, the posterior zygapophyseal joints enlarge to develop osteophytes, the intervertebral disc becomes fibrotic and traction spurs may develop on the anterior and/or posterior aspect of the vertebral body, occasionally leading to spontaneous fusion (Figs 8.22, 8.23). These changes occur during the third stage of the degenerative process, stabilization, and the patient is often painfree (as well as hypomobile) (Kirkaldy-Willis 1983). The risk at this stage is the development of fixed central and/or lateral

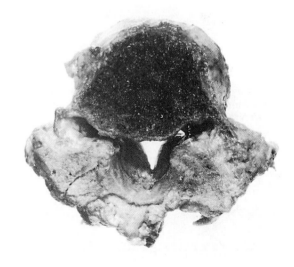

Figure 8.22   Macroscopic transverse section of the L5–S1 segment illustrating fixed central and lateral stenosis. The central and lateral canals are markedly narrowed by osteophytosis. (Reproduced with permission from Kirkaldy-Willis 1983.)

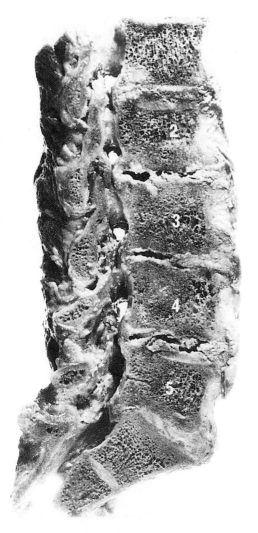

Figure 8.23 Macroscopic sagittal section of the lumbar spine illustrating multilevel spinal stenosis. (Reproduced with permission from Kirkaldy-Willis 1983.)

stenosis due to osseous trespass on the spinal canal and/or lateral recess with attendant peripheral symptoms of neurogenic vascular claudication (Sunderland 1978).

Treatment of segmental instability at the lumbosacral junction

Treatment of the lumbosacral junction forms part of the overall rehabilitation of the lumbo-pelvic-hip complex. The ultimate goal is to restore the ability to control and transfer forces through the trunk to the lower extremity, and this requires stabilization of L5–S1. The following section outlines the therapy indicated during the substrate and the fibroblastic stage of repair when localized hypermobility of L5–S1 is found.

The myofascial components of therapy (restoration of the force closure mechanism) are crucial to the rehabilitation of the hypermobile lumbosacral junction and will be discussed in Chapter 11.

Substrate phase

During the first 4 to 6 days after injury, the goal of treatment is hemostasis of the wound. At home, the frequent application of ice together with rest is the treatment of choice.

Fibroblastic phase

With the resolution of active range of movement, the hypermobile lumbosacral junction becomes apparent. During this stage of repair, treatment is dependent upon which tissues have lost their kinetic ability and upon whether or not neurological impedance has occurred.

If used at all, specific mobilization techniques must be carefully applied and kept well within the physiological range of motion since it is stability, not mobility, that is required. Some clinicians use mobilization techniques as analgesic tools (e.g. for the neurophysiological effects of large afferent fiber stimulation on nociception); however, the electrotherapeutic modalities available today serve the same purpose. Ultrasound should be given at this stage for its influence on collagen production. Clinically, it appears that laser can be an effective treatment at this time.

If impedance of the motor and/or sensory nerve roots is present, intermittent mechanical traction is indicated. The poundage required is that which is necessary to separate the joint, and the usual treatment time is 15 minutes with hold and rest periods of 10 seconds each. The neurological tests as well as the neural mobility tests are used as the objective guides to the success of the treatment and should be monitored before and after each treatment session.

The tests for stability to compression, torsion and shear are repeated frequently to assess the patient's progress. However, if the degree of trauma and subsequent kinetic decompensation has been significant, progress will be slow since the restoration of kinetic function requires 6 to 18 months of healing time (see Ch. 6). During this time, or if the loss of kinetic strength is permanent (Kirkaldy-Willis (1983) stage 2, instability phase, of the degenerative process), stabilization exercises and ergonomic retraining become the crux of therapy (see Ch. 11).

NORMAL MOBILITY WITH PAIN

Rotation sprains are most commonly seen at the L4–L5 segment since the iliolumbar ligament protects the lumbosacral junction against rotational trauma (Bogduk 1997, Taylor et al 1990, Twomey et al 1989)). However, this ligament ties the L5 vertebra directly to the adjacent innominate which increases the risk of secondary breakdown as a consequence of altered function of the pelvic girdle.

Clinically, the patient presents with localized pain at the lumbosacral junction which is easily exacerbated by palpation. However, careful objective evaluation of mobility reveals normal kinematic and kinetic function. The only biomechanical cause for this dysfunction is overuse of the articular and myofascial tissues in compensation for altered function elsewhere. Although local treatment may be required for pain reduction, correction of the global lumbo-pelvic-hip biomechanics is necessary for the prevention of recurrence. Alternatively, the patient may have a disorder which is not biomechanical in nature, a possibility of which the clinician must always be aware.

Box 8.2 Case history

A 38-year-old carpenter presented at the clinic 3 weeks after the recurrence of low back pain. He had experienced multiple episodes of lumbosacral pain in the past, some of which had required time off work and medical attention. This episode developed following a 12-hour drive which had necessitated prolonged periods of sitting in a kyphotic position. Over the next 3 weeks, the local lumbosacral pain had spread distally into the right buttock, posterior thigh and leg to the mid-calf. Dysaesthesia was not reported. The major aggravating factors included forward bending and sitting in kyphosis. Walking and rest both afforded some relief.

Objectively, during forward bending of the trunk a reversed lumbo-pelvic pattern of motion occurred such that the lumbar spine remained extended while the pelvic girdle flexed forward on the femoral heads. Although no support was required during forward bending, the patient returned to erect standing by supporting the weight of his trunk with his hands on his thighs.

Arthrokinetically, both the local and the referred pain were easily reproduced with a passive compression stress test as well as passive torsion to the right. The neural mobility of the L4 to S1 nerve roots was restricted to 45° by pain and reactive hamstring muscle spasm. The clinical neurological tests were normal for both motor and sensory conductivity.

As resolution occurred and specific stability testing was possible, segmental instability of L5–S1 was revealed. The degree of anteroposterior translation was excessive and the end feel of motion less firm than the segments above. This is a common pattern of presentation of the patient who, without appropriate care, initially presents without 'hard' neurological signs and is definitely at risk for future episodes of low back pain given the loss of segmental stability.

Treatment in the early stages included electrotherapeutic analgesic modalities for pain reduction and intermittent mechanical traction aimed at restoring the neural mobility. Stabilization retraining through exercise (Ch. 11) was the focus of therapy.

9

The pelvic girdle: clinical syndromes

HISTORY

At the beginning of the twentieth century, practitioners believed that the sacroiliac joint was the major source of sciatica, admitting that, as well as sciatica, 'lumbago [and] backache ... were frequently caused by an abnormal amount of motion in the pelvic joints, especially the sacroiliac synchondrosis' (Meisenbach 1911). Aside from trauma, the influence of poor posture and also lumbo-pelvic adaptation to extrinsic factors were recognized as being integral to the etiology of decompensation.

The etiology of the pelvic girdle dysfunction is not always clear, but there are many features of definite importance. At times, the lesion apparently represents simply an excess of a normal physiological process. At other times, trauma is a definite factor, 'sitting down hard', or the 'giving way' under severe strains, such as lifting, being the two most common forms of injury. Attitudes or postures are also of importance in causing or predisposing to joint weakness or displacement (Goldthwait & Osgood 1905).

The causes of mechanical pelvic girdle dysfunction remain the same today. Aside from mechanical trauma, there are a number of conditions which can affect the pelvic girdle secondary to systemic disease. The majority of these are listed in Table 9.1. The reader is referred to Bellamy et al (1983) for a concise description of the conditions tabulated.

In the early twentieth century, sacroiliac joint dysfunction was treated in one of two ways— manipulation or immobilization (Albee 1909,

Table 9.1 Conditions affecting the sacroiliac joint (Bellamy et al 1983)

Inflammatory disorders
Ankylosing spondylitis
Reiter's syndrome
Inflammatory bowel disease
Psoriatic spondylitis
Rheumatoid arthritis
Juvenile rheumatoid arthritis
Pustulotic arthro-osteitis
Familial Mediterranean fever
Behçet's syndrome
Relapsing polychondritis
Whipple's disease

Joint infection
Pyogenic
Brucellosis
Tuberculosis

Metabolic disorders
Gout
Calcium pyrophosphate deposition disease
Hyperparathyroidism

Miscellaneous
Osteitis condensans ilii
Paget's disease
Acro-osteolysis, in polyvinyl chloride workers
Alkaptonuria
Gaucher's disease
Tuberous sclerosis

Fryette 1914, Goldthwait & Osgood 1905, Meisenbach 1911, Young 1940). The manipulation techniques for the 'subluxed' sacroiliac joints are poorly described in the literature and usually include non-specific pressure over the sacrum.

The correction of the subluxation may be brought about in several ways. At times simply hyperextending the spine considerably by having the patient lie with a firm pillow under the 'hollow of the back', may, by raising the lumbar spine, draw the sacrum into place. At other times the same thing may be accomplished by having the patient lie face downward with the thighs and legs supported upon one table, the head and shoulders upon another, the body hanging entirely unsupported between. In this position the weight of the body drags the spine forward, which favors the replacement of the sacrum. If this is successful the plaster jacket which is to hold the spine and the pelvic joints may be applied before the patient is moved (Goldthwait & Osgood 1905).

In principle, treatment of the pelvic girdle remains unchanged. Hypomobile joints are mobilized whereas unstable joints (those with impaired load transfer) are stabilized. The goal of therapy is to restore the optimal biomechanics via mobilization techniques and exercise programs. The soft tissues about the pelvic girdle are treated according to the presenting stage of repair (i.e. substrate, fibroblastic, maturation) which has been covered in detail in Chapter 6 and outlined in Chapter 8 under treatment of the hypomobile lumbosacral junction and will not be discussed again here. This chapter will outline the specific mobilization techniques used to restore mobility to the stiff sacroiliac joint, and the manipulation techniques used to reduce excessive compression of the sacroiliac joint.

The myofascial components of therapy (restoration of the force closure mechanism) will be discussed in Chapter 11.

CLASSIFICATION

The classifications for mechanical dysfunction within the pelvic girdle are multiple and usually describe restricted osteokinematic function of either the sacrum or the innominate. Subsequently, labels such as 'posterior innominate', 'anterior sacrum', 'forward sacral torsion' and 'upslips' have emerged with little regard to universal nomenclature. The difficulty with this method of classification arises when interdisciplinary communication is attempted.

For the clinician, classifications which follow a biomechanical model based on mobility and stability of the articular structures have proven more useful in facilitating a consistent approach to treatment and can be easily communicated. In keeping with this model, articular dysfunction of the pelvic girdle can be classified into three groups, each of which describes the objective findings noted on mobility/stability testing and suggests the appropriate therapy. They include:

1. hypomobility with or without pain
2. hypermobility/instability with or without pain
3. normal mobility with pain.

This classification pertains to the arthrokinematic and arthrokinetic function of the sacroiliac joint/pubic symphysis. This classification does not provide a specific anatomical cause for the aberrant mobility noted; however, since mobilization and stabilization techniques used in manual therapy are specific to restoring movement patterns, definition of the cause is not always required for formulating treatment plans.

HYPOMOBILITY WITH OR WITHOUT PAIN

Subjective findings

Symptoms from a hypomobile sacroiliac joint may develop insidiously or suddenly. There is usually an element of trauma in the history; typically, a fall on the buttocks or a lifting incident has occurred some time in the past. By the time the sacroiliac joint has become stiff, the substrate and fibroblastic phase of healing have passed. Acutely sprained sacroiliac joints are painful, but not hypomobile, and are treated in the manner outlined for the lumbosacral junction (Ch. 8).

Sacroiliac joint pain is usually localized to the region around the joint (Fortin et al 1997); however, it may radiate through the pelvis to the anterior aspect of the ipsilateral groin and/or down the posterolateral buttock and thigh to the knee. When the hypomobility has been long standing, the site of pain may switch to the contralateral side. The soft tissue and ligaments surrounding the stiff joint may be a source of nociception, although inconsistencies are common. Dysaesthesia is not often reported. The aggravating activities commonly include walking, stair climbing/descent, rolling over in bed, getting in/out of chair/car and standing on one leg. These patients are often uncomfortable in any one position or doing any activity for a prolonged period of time and require frequent alterations in posture for relief. Although rest usually affords relief, asymmetric sleeping postures are often more comfortable.

Objective findings

The essential objective finding for classification here is *decreased*, but not blocked, motion of the sacroiliac joint (Fig. 7.28c).

Gait

The normal lumbopelvic rhythm of gait is altered when the sacroiliac joint is hypomobile. The pelvis moves as a unit between the lumbar spine and the legs with less intra-pelvic motion through both the swing and stance phase.

Posture

There is no consistent posture which identifies the hypomobile sacroiliac joint. The innominate on the side of the hypomobility tends to posture toward anterior rotation although posterior rotation patterns have been found.

Functional tests

In the presence of unilateral hypomobility, forward and backward bending of the trunk produces intra-pelvic torsion of the pelvic girdle. This is felt as asymmetrical motion of the PSISs during forward/backward bending. Lateral bending of the trunk can be restricted such that the pelvic girdle does not translate in the coronal plane without deviation.

The hypomobile sacroiliac joint will also affect the ipsilateral rotation tests (both posterior and anterior). The restriction becomes apparent as a reduction or total absence of relative motion between the innominate and the sacrum. The supine and prone active straight leg raise tests are performed without difficulty.

Articular mobility/stability tests

The specific mobility tests for inferoposterior and anterosuperior glide (Ch. 7) reveal the articular restriction. Both directions are commonly reduced when the sacroiliac joint is hypomobile. This appears to be the capsular pattern of restriction for this joint. The stability tests for anteroposterior and superoinferior translation (Ch. 7) confirm the reduction in joint play. The provocation of pain on mobility/stability and stress testing (Ch. 7) depends on the stage of pathology, the nature of the injury and the degree of inflammation present at the time of examination. The pain patterns are highly variable and inconsistent (Dreyfuss et al 1996).

Muscle function tests

Alterations in muscle balance and function are present when the sacroiliac joint is hypomobile. The patterns of presentation are multiple and variable. The treatment approach to muscle function is addressed in Chapter 11.

Neurological tests

Impedance of neurological function and/or dural mobility can occur, and depends on the degree of decompensation of the lumbosacral junction as a consequence of the hypomobile sacroiliac joint.

Treatment of the hypomobile sacroiliac joint

When the regional muscles become tight (e.g. piriformis, hamstrings), the mobility of the pelvic girdle (innominate or sacrum) can be affected; however, the sacroiliac joint itself remains mobile. This is why it is imperative to evaluate the mobility of the joint with tests which do not involve active contraction or passive lengthening of the muscles. When the myofascial system is the primary source of dysfunction, specific muscle-lengthening techniques can be effective in restoring the osteokinematics of the pelvic girdle. These techniques are often referred to as 'muscle energy' techniques or active mobilization techniques. They facilitate the restoration of motion at the sacroiliac joint and can be used in conjunction with the passive mobilization technique.

Passive mobilization for restricted inferoposterior glide of innominate on sacrum

The patient is supine, with the hips and knees flexed. With the long and ring finger of one hand, palpate the sacral sulcus just medial to the PSIS (Fig. 7.25). With the index finger of the same hand, palpate the lumbosacral junction. With the

heel of the other hand, palpate the ipsilateral ASIS and the iliac crest. Apply a grade 2 to 4 anterior rotation force (Fig. 9.1) to the innominate to produce an inferoposterior glide at the sacroiliac joint (Lee & Walsh 1996). This glide is also associated with counternutation of the sacrum. The sacroiliac joint may be mobilized through the sacrum by applying a grade 2 to 4 counternutation force to the apex of the sacrum (Fig. 9.2) (Lee & Walsh 1996).

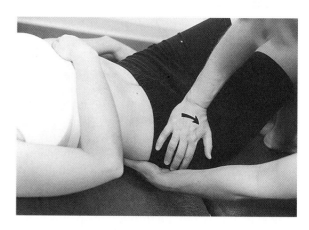

Figure 9.1 Passive mobilization for the sacroiliac joint, using anterior rotation of the innominate to restore the inferoposterior glide of the innominate relative to the sacrum (same motion as anterosuperior glide of the sacrum relative to the innominate) (Lee & Walsh 1996).

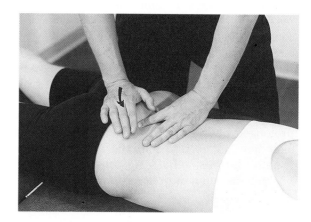

Figure 9.2 Passive mobilization technique for the sacroiliac joint, using counternutation of the sacrum to restore the anterosuperior glide of the sacrum relative to the innominate (same motion as inferoposterior glide of the innominate relative to the sacrum) (Lee & Walsh 1996).

Active mobilization for restricted inferoposterior glide of innominate on sacrum (restricted anterior rotation)

With the patient prone, lying close to the edge of the table, the anterior aspect of the distal thigh is palpated with the caudal hand, while the PSIS of the innominate is palpated with the heel of the cranial hand.

The limit of anterior rotation of the innominate is reached by passively extending the femur with the caudal hand and applying an anterior rotation force to the innominate with the cranial hand (Fig. 9.3) (Lee & Walsh 1996). From this position, the patient is instructed to resist further hip extension which is gently increased by the therapist. The isometric contraction is held for up to 5 seconds followed by a period of complete relaxation. The innominate is then passively taken to the new barrier of anterior rotation. The technique is repeated three times followed by re-evaluation of function.

Home exercise

Unilateral hip extension exercises in the prone position are given to augment the mobilization techniques.

Passive mobilization for restricted anterosuperior glide of innominate on sacrum

The patient is supine with their hips and knees flexed. With the long and ring finger of one hand, palpate the sacral sulcus just medial to the PSIS (Fig. 7.25). With the index finger of the same hand, palpate the lumbosacral junction. With the heel of the other hand, palpate the ipsilateral ASIS and the iliac crest. Apply a grade 2 to 4 posterior rotation force (Fig. 9.4) (Lee & Walsh 1996) to the innominate to produce an anterosuperior glide at the sacroiliac joint. This glide is also associated with nutation of the sacrum. The sacroiliac joint may be mobilized through the sacrum by applying a grade 2 to 4 nutation force to the base of the sacrum (Fig. 9.5) (Lee & Walsh 1996).

Active mobilization for restricted anterosuperior glide of innominate on sacrum (restricted posterior rotation)

With the patient supine, lying close to the edge of the table, the ischial tuberosity is palpated with the caudal hand (Fig. 9.6) (Lee & Walsh 1996). The flexed hip and knee are supported against the therapist's shoulder and arm. The

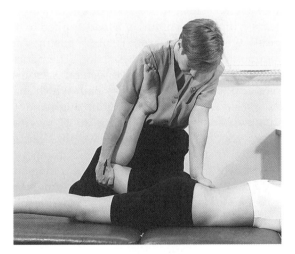

Figure 9.3 Active mobilization technique to restore anterior rotation of the innominate and the inferoposterior glide of the innominate relative to the sacrum (Lee & Walsh 1996).

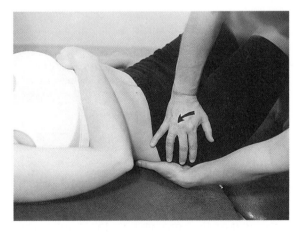

Figure 9.4 Passive mobilization for the sacroiliac joint, using posterior rotation of the innominate to restore the anterosuperior glide of the innominate relative to the sacrum (same motion as inferoposterior glide of the sacrum relative to the innominate) (Lee & Walsh 1996).

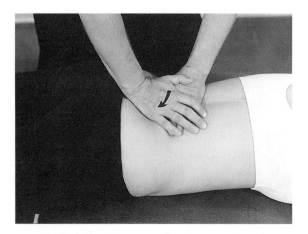

Figure 9.5 Passive mobilization technique for the sacroiliac joint, using nutation of the sacrum to restore the inferoposterior glide of the sacrum relative to the innominate (same motion as anterosuperior glide of the innominate relative to the sacrum) (Lee & Walsh 1996).

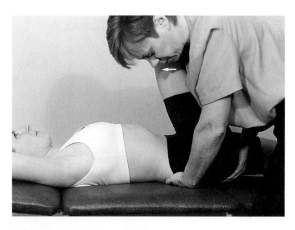

Figure 9.6 Active mobilization technique to restore posterior rotation of the innominate and the anterosuperior glide of the innominate relative to the sacrum (Lee & Walsh 1996).

index and long fingers of the other hand palpate the lumbosacral junction and the sacral sulcus to ensure localization of the technique.

The limit of posterior rotation of the innominate is reached by passively flexing the femur until motion is perceived at the lumbosacral junction. The motion barrier for the sacroiliac joint has then been reached. From this position, the patient is instructed to resist further hip flexion which is gently increased by the

therapist. The isometric contraction is held for up to 5 seconds, followed by a period of complete relaxation. The innominate is then passively taken to the new barrier of posterior rotation. The technique is repeated three times followed by re-evaluation of function.

Home exercise

Unilateral hip flexion exercises in the supine position are given to augment the mobilization techniques.

HYPERMOBILITY/INSTABILITY WITH OR WITHOUT PAIN

Hypermobility/instability of the sacroiliac joint girdle can occur following repeated micro-trauma, one major trauma or secondary to hormonal changes such as those associated with pregnancy (see Ch. 5). The essential objective finding for classification here is *increased* motion of the sacroiliac joint coupled with a soft end feel on stability testing (Ch. 7. Fig. 7.28b).

Subjective findings

The mode of onset is usually sudden. An unexpected vertical load through a weight-bearing limb (or ischium) or a load applied to the trunk while in a flexed/rotated posture are common causes of this dysfunction. The patient reports a sudden onset of unilateral sacroiliac joint and/or pubic symphysis pain which may radiate into the buttock, posterior thigh and/or abdomen and groin. The aggravating activities commonly include unilateral weight-bearing, bending forward, lifting, lying supine and rolling over from this position, fast walking and any activity for prolonged periods of time. Rest usually affords relief as long as the irritable joint is not under stress while in the resting position.

Objective findings

If the injuring force is sufficient to significantly irritate the articular structures, there can be a massive muscle response which holds the sacroiliac joint at the limit of its physiological range. If the force has stretched the passive restraints, the joint may be held slightly beyond its usual physiological range. In the past, this dysfunction has been called a subluxation or fixation (Lee 1997b).

In every instance, the mobility and stability (joint play) tests are totally blocked, and the positional findings of the innominate and/or sacrum differentiate the various dysfunctions. The treatment technique must involve reduction of articular compression if symmetry is to be restored to the pelvic girdle.

The joint appears to be hypomobile and the underlying articular instability cannot be determined until the articular compression is reduced. Vertical forces through the innominate or the leg stress the passive restraints in the craniocaudal plane and the resultant position of the innominate is superior in either anterior (more commonly) or posterior rotation. If the individual has very good form closure and is able to resist the vertical force, the dysfunction may only have a rotary component (anterior or posterior innominate rotation) in the presence of excessive articular compression.

Horizontal translation forces through the trunk stress the passive restraints in the anteroposterior plane and the resultant position of the sacrum is either anterior (towards nutation) or posterior (towards counternutation) translation. The excessive approximation of the articular structures together with the altered position of the innominate/sacrum distorts the afferent input to the motor control system significantly altering the efficiency of the load transfer system.

Gait

The displacement of the center of gravity is exaggerated when the sacroiliac joint is unstable or excessively compressed. The patient attempts to compensate for the lack of stability by reducing the shear forces through the sacroiliac joint. In the compensated gait pattern, the patient transfers his or her weight laterally over the involved limb (compensated Trendelenburg sign), thus reducing the vertical shear forces through the joint (Lee 1997) (Fig. 5.41). In the non-compensated gait pattern, the patient tends to demonstrate a true Trendelenburg sign. The pelvic girdle abducts excessively (on the unstable weight-bearing side) (Fig. 5.42). The femur abducts relative to the foot, thus bringing the center of gravity closer to the sacroiliac joint and reduces the vertical shear force.

Posture

In standing and sitting, the patient tends to adopt a resting posture which unloads the affected sacroiliac joint.

Functional tests

When the sacroiliac joint is excessively compressed, the pattern of presentation on functional testing is similar to that of a hypomobile sacroiliac joint. Asymmetry of motion of the PSISs occurs on both forward and backward bending of the trunk and the ability to laterally translate the pelvic girdle in the coronal plane during lateral bending is restricted. The ipsilateral rotation tests (posterior/anterior) in standing are blocked when the joint is compressed. The supine and prone active straight leg raise tests are poorly performed and often painful. When form closure is augmented in the presence of excessive articular compression, the ability to actively straight leg raise does not improve and may get worse.

If the joint is unstable and not excessively compressed (Fig. 7.28b), augmenting form closure with manual compression of the sacroiliac joint (Ch. 7) results in improved function during this test. When force closure is augmented in the presence of excessive articular compression, the ability to actively straight leg raise does not improve. If the joint is unstable and not excessively compressed, augmenting the force closure mechanism through the anterior and posterior sling of the outer unit results in improved function during this test.

Articular mobility/stability tests

The specific mobility tests for inferoposterior and anterosuperior glide (Ch. 7) are completely blocked when the unstable sacroiliac joint is excessively compressed. The distinguishing feature between the compressed joint and the hypomobile joint is the quality of the end feel on mobility/stability testing. The compressed joint has no give at the end of the range and a very hard sensation is encountered as soon as the test begins. In addition, the resting position of the innominates/sacrum (see positional findings in the specific lesions) is very asymmetric. The stability tests for anteroposterior and supero-inferior translation (Ch. 7) are also blocked when the unstable joint is excessively compressed. The stability tests reveal increased motion and a very soft end feel when the unstable joint is not overly compressed. The direction of the instability depends on the force applied to the joint at the time of injury (see specific lesions). The provocation of pain on mobility/stability and stress testing (Ch. 7) depends on the stage of pathology, the nature of the injury and the degree of inflammation present at the time of examination. The pain patterns are highly variable and inconsistent (Dreyfuss et al 1996).

Muscle function tests

Disruption of the sacroiliac joint has a dramatic and immediate influence on muscle function. The gluteii appear to be particularly inhibited when the sacroiliac joint is excessively compressed. Isolation of the pelvic floor, the transversus abdominis, gluteus maximus and medius is often difficult until the compression is reduced. The function of the inner and outer unit of muscles (Ch. 5) is crucial to successful rehabilitation of the unstable pelvic girdle and forms the basis of treatment (Ch. 11).

Nerve function tests

It is not uncommon to see loss of function of the L5 and S1 nerve roots when the sacroiliac joint has been compressed in asymmetry for some time. The loss of mobility of the sacroiliac joint, coupled with the altered position of the sacrum and the loss of support from the sacrotuberous ligament and/or iliolumbar ligament for the lumbosacral junction, can rapidly lead to decompensation of the intervertebral disc. Central and/or lateral protrusions/herniations of the lumbosacral disc can interfere directly with the emerging nerve roots or compromise the nerve's vascular supply.

Treatment of the compressed sacroiliac joint

Compression: innominate superior and anteriorly rotated

This dysfunction occurs when a vertical force posterior to the axis of sacroiliac joint motion exceeds the joint's resistance (Fig. 9.7). On positional testing, the innominate is anteriorly rotated on the side of the lesion and the ischial tuberosity is superior rendering the ipsilateral sacrotuberous ligament slack. The L5 vertebra and the sacrum are slightly rotated towards the contralateral side. Figure 9.8 illustrates the

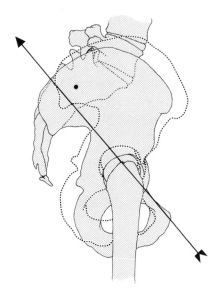

Figure 9.7 The sacroiliac joint can be excessively compressed when a strong vertical force posterior to the axis of rotation (dot) displaces the innominate superiorly in anterior rotation (heavy dotted line).

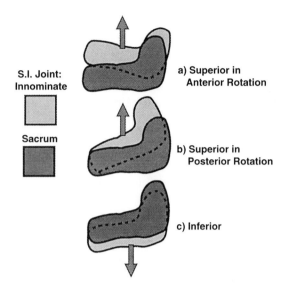

S.I. Joint:
Innominate

Sacrum

a) Superior in
Anterior Rotation

b) Superior in
Posterior Rotation

c) Inferior

Figure 9.8 The direction of the force applied to the sacroiliac joint and the hypothetical displacement against which the muscle system responds in a vertical loading injury.

direction of force applied to the sacroiliac joint and the hypothetical displacement against which the muscle system is responding to produce the excessive compression. Both the mobility and stability tests are completely blocked prior to manipulation.

To reduce the compression, the following technique is used (Fig. 9.9) (Lee & Walsh 1996).

The patient is prone. The therapist grasps the lower leg, proximal to the talocrural joint, on the side to be manipulated. The hip joint is extended and medially rotated such that the line of the femur corresponds to the degree of anterior rotation of the innominate. The motion barrier is reached by applying a longitudinal pull through the leg. A high-velocity, low-amplitude tug is applied through the leg to the sacroiliac joint. A second therapist may assist by stabilizing the inferolateral aspect of the sacrum with the heel of one hand.

After the compression is reduced, the stability tests reveal an excessive superior glide of the sacroiliac joint. The pelvic girdle is then supported with a proper belt (Fig. 9.10) which should be worn just above the greater trochanters. This augments the form and force closure mechanism until such time as the connective tissue tightens and rehabilitation for the force closure mechanism (Ch. 11) is instituted.

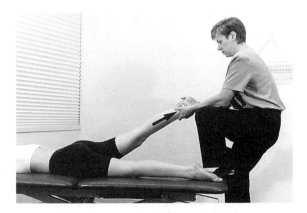

Figure 9.9 High-velocity, low-amplitude thrust technique used to decompress the sacroiliac joint when the innominate is held superiorly in anterior rotation (Lee & Walsh 1996).

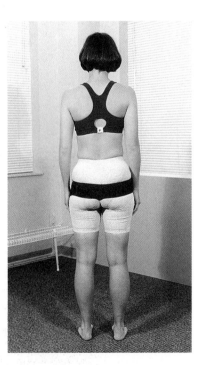

Figure 9.10 After reduction, form closure of the pelvic girdle is augmented with a belt which should be worn just above the greater trochanters. This belt is manufactured by Serola Biomechanics.

Compression: innominate superior and posteriorly rotated

This dysfunction occurs when a vertical force anterior to the axis of sacroiliac joint motion exceeds the joint's resistance (Fig. 9.11). On positional testing, the innominate is posteriorly rotated on the side of the lesion and the ischial tuberosity is superior. The posterior rotation of the innominate coupled with a slight superior translation makes the sacrotuberous ligament tension feel normal. The L5 vertebra and the sacrum are slightly rotated towards the dysfunctional side. Figure 9.8 illustrates the direction of force applied to the sacroiliac joint and the hypothetical displacement against which the muscle system is responding to produce the excessive compression. Both the mobility and stability tests are completely blocked prior to manipulation.

To reduce the compression, the technique described for the superior fixation of the innominate in anterior rotation is modified slightly. The patient is supine. The therapist grasps the

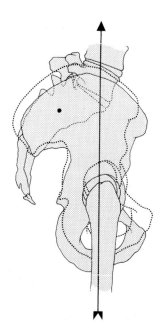

Figure 9.11 The sacroiliac joint can be excessively compressed when a strong vertical force anterior to the axis of rotation (dot) displaces the innominate superior in posterior rotation (heavy dotted line).

lower leg, proximal to the talocrural joint, on the side to be manipulated. The hip joint is flexed and medially rotated such that the line of the femur corresponds to the degree of posterior rotation of the innominate. The motion barrier is reached by applying a longitudinal pull through the leg. A high-velocity, low-amplitude tug is applied through the leg to the sacroiliac joint.

After the compression is reduced, the stability tests reveal an excessive superior glide of the sacroiliac joint. The pelvic girdle is then supported with a proper belt (Fig. 9.10) which should be worn just above the greater trochanters. This augments the form and force closure mechanism until such time as the connective tissue tightens and rehabilitation for the force closure mechanism (Ch. 11) is instituted.

Compression: innominate inferior

This dysfunction is not common, but can occur when a longitudinal traction force occurs down the lower extremity. Getting a foot caught in a ladder or stirrups while falling is one mechanism of injury. The side of the joint restriction on mobility testing identifies the side of the lesion. Positional testing of the innominate confirms the downward position of the innominate relative to the sacrum.

To reduce the compression, the patient is supine with the hip fully flexed on the restricted side (Fig. 9.12) (Lee & Walsh 1996). The therapist grasps the opposite leg, proximal to the talocrural joint. The hip joint is flexed and medially rotated. The motion barrier is reached by applying a caudal pull. A high-velocity, low-amplitude tug is applied through the leg to the contralateral sacroiliac joint. The inferior pull of the innominate is transferred to the sacrum. Its descent provides a superior force to the contralateral innominate thus reducing the compression. Follow-up care is the same as for the previous dysfunctions.

Compression: innominate posteriorly rotated

The mode of onset is usually traumatic, commonly a rotary force through the leg. Often, the

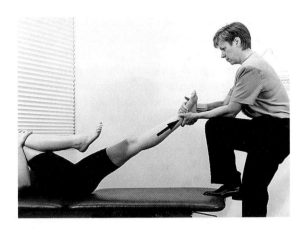

Figure 9.12 High-velocity, low-amplitude thrust technique used to decompress the sacroiliac joint when the right innominate is held inferiorly (Lee & Walsh 1996).

patient reports that one leg slipped out from under them, or that they stepped unexpectedly off a kerb. An overzealous kick against a missed target is another frequent etiology. The pure rotation dysfunctions of the innominate with an excessive compression of the sacroiliac joint have a marked impact on gait. Both the stance and the swing phases are shortened and the patient hobbles into the clinic. When the sacroiliac joint is overly compressed and the innominate is held in posterior rotation, the ASIS is superior, the PSIS is inferior, the ischial tuberosities are level and the sacrotuberous ligament is under marked tension on the restricted side. The L5 vertebra as well as the sacrum tends to be rotated towards the side of the dysfunction.

To reduce the compression, the following technique is used. With the patient prone, lying close to the edge of the table, the anterior aspect of the distal thigh is palpated with the caudal hand, while the PSIS of the innominate is palpated with the heel of the cranial hand.

The limit of anterior rotation of the innominate is reached by passively extending the femur with the caudal hand and applying an anterolateral force to the innominate with the cranial hand (Fig. 9.3). From this position, a high-velocity, low-amplitude thrust is applied through the innominate in an anterolateral direction while the other hand simultaneously extends the femur, thus anteriorly rotating the innominate. The lateral pressure on the PSIS distracts the posterior aspect of the sacroiliac joint. Re-evaluation of the mobility/stability tests confirms the success of the technique. The degree of instability in the vertical plane is less than that found in the superior lesions. Follow-up care however, is the same.

Compression: innominate anteriorly rotated

The mechanism of injury is traumatic with hyperextension of the leg being a significant factor. On positional testing, the ASIS is inferior, PSIS superior, ischial tuberosities are level and the sacrotuberous ligament still palpable but less taut than normal on the side of the dysfunction. The L5 vertebra and the sacrum tend to rotate away from the affected side.

To decompress the joint, the following technique is used. With the patient supine lying in left side flexion, the arms are crossed to opposite shoulders and the right leg is crossed over the left at the ankles. The therapist stands facing the patient's right side. Rotate the thoracolumbar spine to the right and fix the lumbosacral junction with the cranial hand/arm. Palpate the left ASIS and iliac crest with the caudal hand. With the caudal hand, apply a high-velocity, low-amplitude posterior lateral force to the innominate while stabilizing the L5 and sacrum. The lateral pressure on the ASIS distracts the anterior aspect of the sacroiliac joint. Re-evaluation of the mobility/stability tests confirms the success of the technique. The degree of instability in the vertical plane is less than that found in the superior lesions. Follow-up care however, is the same.

Compression: sacrum anterior

The mode of onset is traumatic, usually a lifting injury associated with a twist. The patient often reports hearing and feeling a pop and a sharp pain localized to the sacroiliac joint at the time of the injury. On positional testing, the sacral base is anterior on the side of the articular restriction and this displacement persists in all positions of the trunk — hyperflexion, neutral and hyperextension. Relative to S1, the L5 vertebra is rotated towards the side of the dysfunction. Figure 9.13 illustrates the direction of force applied to the sacroiliac joint and the hypothetical displacement against which the muscle system is responding to produce the excessive compression. Both the mobility and stability tests are completely blocked prior to manipulation.

To decompress the right sacroiliac joint, the following technique is used (Fig. 9.14) (Lee & Walsh 1996). With the patient in right side-lying

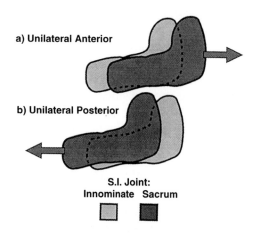

a) Unilateral Anterior

b) Unilateral Posterior

S.I. Joint:
Innominate   Sacrum

Figure 9.13 The direction of the force applied to the sacroiliac joint and the hypothetical displacement against which the muscle system responds in a horizontal translation loading injury.

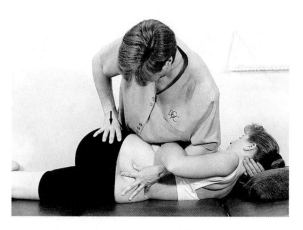

Figure 9.14 High velocity, low amplitude thrust technique used to decompress the sacroiliac joint when the sacrum is held anterior at the right sacroiliac joint (Lee & Walsh 1996).

and the lower leg extended and the upper hip and knee flexed, the thoracolumbar spine is rotated until L5–S1 is felt to be fully rotated to the left. The lateral aspect of the spinous process of the L5 vertebra is firmly stabilized with one thumb to maintain the rotation at the lumbosacral junction. With the other hand, the left innominate and the lumbosacral unit are rotated to the right *about a pure vertical axis through the pelvic girdle* to the motion barrier allowing the table to stabilize the right innominate. From this position, a high-velocity, low-amplitude thrust is applied through the left innominate and the sacrum to produce distraction of the posterior aspect of the sacroiliac joint and posterior translation of the right sacral base relative to the right innominate. Following decompression of the joint, the stability tests are repeated. In this instance, an increase in anteroposterior translation (Fig. 9.13) will be palpated on the right. The pelvic girdle is then supported with a proper belt (Fig. 9.10) which should be worn just above the greater trochanters. This augments the form and force closure mechanism until such time as the connective tissue tightens and rehabilitation for the force closure mechanism (Ch. 11) is instituted.

Compression: sacrum posterior

The mechanism of injury and clinical presentation is identical to that of the anterior translation lesion. On positional testing, the sacral base is posterior on the side of the articular restriction and this displacement persists in all positions of the trunk—hyperflexion, neutral and hyperextension. Relative to S1, the L5 vertebra is rotated away from the side of the dysfunction. Figure 9.13 illustrates the direction of the force applied to the sacroiliac joint and the hypothetical displacement against which the muscle system is responding to produce the excessive compression. Both the mobility and stability tests are completely blocked prior to manipulation.

To decompress the right sacroiliac joint, the following technique is used (Fig. 9.15) (Lee & Walsh 1996). With the patient prone and the right

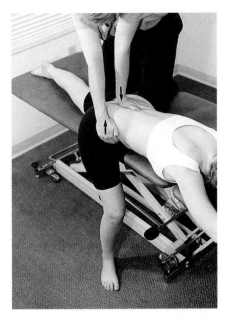

Figure 9.15 High-velocity, low-amplitude thrust technique used to decompress the sacroiliac joint when the sacrum is held posterior at the right sacroiliac joint (Lee & Walsh 1996).

hip and knee flexed over the side of the table, the right sacral base is palpated with the heel of the left hand. With the other hand, the right iliac crest and the ASIS are palpated. A posterior glide is applied to the innominate against the fixed sacrum. When the motion barrier has been reached, a high-velocity, low-amplitude thrust is applied to the sacrum in an anterior direction. Following decompression of the joint, the stability tests are repeated. In this instance, an increase in anteroposterior translation (Fig. 9.13) will be palpated on the right. The pelvic girdle is then supported with a proper belt (Fig. 9.10) which should be worn just above the greater

trochanters. This augments the form and force closure mechanism until such time as the connective tissue tightens and rehabilitation for the force closure mechanism (Ch. 11) is instituted.

On occasion, the degree of loss of form closure is such that the muscle system is not able to stabilize the pelvic girdle in weight-bearing activities. In this situation, prolotherapy (Dorman 1994, 1997) can be a valuable aid in the restoration of form closure. The ligaments of the sacroiliac joint are injected with a solution which promotes the synthesis of collagen by the fibroblasts. During a course of prolotherapy (usually 3 months), the specific stability tests of the sacroiliac joint can be felt to improve. In other words, the quantity of translation becomes reduced and the end feel becomes firmer. Once form closure has been re-established, stabilization therapy through exercise (Ch. 11) can begin.

NORMAL MOBILITY WITH PAIN

Patients presenting with localized pain within the pelvic girdle in the absence of positive mobility/stability findings can be challenging to treat. The only cause of a biomechanical nature for this can be overuse of the articular and myofascial tissues secondary to altered function elsewhere (hip, knee, foot). Treating the pain with analgesic modalities and manual techniques affords temporary relief at best. A biomechanical approach to evaluation and treatment is the best way to improve function with these patients. Alternatively, the patient may have a disorder which is not biomechanical in nature (see Table 9.1), a possibility of which the clinician must always be aware.

10

The hip: clinical syndromes

Disorders of the hip are not rare; in fact muscle imbalances which affect femoral motion are common even among the young. In addition, and perhaps because of persistent muscle imbalance, degenerative arthrosis of the hip joint can occur very early. Grieve (1983) notes that 'about 10% to 11% of people aged below 30 years have a degree of arthrosis, some with hip involvement.' Restricted femoral motion has a large impact on the function of the pelvic girdle and low back both of which attempt to compensate for the loss of motion at the hip. Over time, symptoms of tissue breakdown within the lumbar spine and pelvic girdle may begin insidiously, secondary to the restriction at the hip. The pain resolves once the biomechanics of the lumbo-pelvic-hip region are restored.

CLASSIFICATION

Hip disorders are commonly classified according to the age group in which they occur (Table 10.1). Alternatively, disorders have been classified as articular or non-articular (Table 10.2).

For the clinician, classifications which follow a biomechanical model based on mobility, bearing in mind the specific disorders relative to the patient's age group, are more useful in facilitating a consistent approach to assessment and treatment. In keeping with this model, disorders of the hip can be classified into two groups, each of which describes the objective findings noted on mobility testing. They include:

Table 10.1 Classification of hip disorders according to age group (Cyriax 1954)

Newborn
Congenital dislocation of the hip

Ages 4–12 years
Perthes' disease
Tuberculosis
Transitory arthritis

Ages 12–17 years
Slipped femoral epiphysis
Osteochondritis dissecans

Young adults
Muscle lesions
Bursitis

Adults
Arthritis
   Osteoarthritis
   Rheumatoid arthritis
   Ankylosing spondylitis
Bursitis
Loose bodies

Table 10.2 Articular vs. non-articular disorders of the hip (Adams 1973)

Articular disorders of the hip
Congenital deformities
   Congenital dislocation of the hip
   Arthritis
   Transient arthritis of children
   Pyogenic arthritis
   Rheumatoid arthritis
   Tuberculous arthritis
   Osteoarthritis
   Ankylosing spondylitis
Osteochondritis
   Perthes' disease (pseudocoxalgia)
Mechanical disorders
   Slipped upper femoral epiphysis
Osteitis deformans (Paget's disease)

Non-articular disorders in the region of the hip
Deformities
   Coxa vara
Infections
   Tuberculosis of the trochanteric bursa

1. hypomobility with or without pain
2. normal mobility with pain.

This classification pertains to the osteokinematic function of the femur relative to the innominate which depends on the arthrokinematic and myokinematic function of the hip. Like those for the lumbosacral junction and the pelvic girdle, this classification does not provide a specific anatomical cause for the aberrant mobility noted; however, it is important to recall that the goal of therapy is to improve functional movement patterns regardless of the underlying diagnosis. The aim of all evaluation procedures is to identify the system (i.e. articular vs. myofascial) which is aberrantly altering the osteokinematic function of the femur during functional movement, so that treatment can be directed accordingly.

HYPOMOBILITY WITH OR WITHOUT PAIN

The hip joint, like all other synovial joints, degenerates slowly and consequently can present a variety of clinical pictures. In the early stages of pathology, altered afferent input from the mechanoreceptors within the joint capsule (see Ch. 4) can adversely affect the perceptual component of static joint position, dynamic proprioception and stability as well as the resting tone of the muscles about the hip joint. The patient may state that the limb feels weak and tends to give way rather than being restricted in range, particularly during athletic endeavors.

'The implications are obvious—if degenerative change has grossly disturbed afferent impulse traffic from capsular mechanoreceptors, the partial loss of the "governor" for joint congruity has increased the susceptibility of such joints to articular strains from normally trivial stress' (Grieve 1983). Thus the degenerative process is facilitated and the muscle imbalance perpetuated.

The essential objective finding for classification here is decreased osteokinematic motion of the femur relative to the innominate bone. The etiology may be either articular or myofascial and is found amongst all age groups.

Subjective findings

In the early stages, a stiff hip due to mild muscle imbalance (eg. tight tensor fascia lata/iliotibial band and weak gluteus medius, tight external rotators and weak internal rotators, tight hip flexors and weak hip extensors) produces symptoms which are usually not local. Even minor restrictions of femoral motion can cause compensatory hypermobility of the sacroiliac joint, the lumbosacral junction and/or the knee/patellofemoral joint, and these articulations are more commonly the source of pain. When trauma is not a factor, the onset of symptoms is insidious.

Compensatory pain from the sacroiliac joint and/or the lumbosacral junction is aggravated by any activity which requires excessive motion from the low back/pelvis in compensation for restrictions of the femur. For example, backward bending of the trunk often elicits pain at the lumbosacral junction when L5–S1 overextends to compensate for restricted femoral extension secondary to a tight or shortened iliopsoas. A painful, long dorsal ligament is aggravated in forward bending of the trunk when tight hamstrings initiate early counternutation of the sacrum through their attachment to the sacrotuberous ligament. The location of pain and the alleviation with local anaesthetic is not often helpful in directing biomechanical treatment. Understanding the biomechanics often explains the cause of local tissue breakdown and subsequently the pain pattern.

When the hip joint itself becomes symptomatic, as in osteoarthritis, the location of pain can be variable. Wroblewski (1978) studied the pain patterns in 89 patients with osteoarthritis of the hip joint, and the variation noted is tabulated in Table 10.3. The hip joint, being derived from the L3 mesoderm, can refer pain anywhere within the L3 dermatome and/or sclerotome. Clinically, it is common to find the primary complaint being *knee* pain, which the patient completely dissociates from 'the usual backache', often denying local hip pain entirely.

With moderate articular degeneration, the aggravating activities include walking, stair climbing/descent and weight bearing in flexion (i.e. squat). In the early stages, more demanding activities such as sport may be required to aggravate the condition.

Table 10.3   Pain patterns in 89 patients with osteoarthritis of the hip joint (From Wroblewski 1978)

Area of pain	Number of patients
Greater trochanter	71
Medial buttock	40
Groin	47
Anterior thigh	63
Knee	70
Shin	40

Objective findings

Gait

Hypomobility of the hip is reflected in the patient's gait pattern. The stance phase is often shortened, thus creating a vertical limp. If the altered mechanoreceptor input from the articular capsule significantly alters the strength of the lateral system (stabilizers of the hip), there will be a loss of dynamic stability (force closure) compensated for by a lateral limp (compensated Trendelenburg sign; Fig. 5.41). The center of gravity deviates laterally in order to reduce the muscle requirements of unilateral stance (see Ch. 5).

Functional tests

When the hip is restricted in flexion/extension unilaterally, full forward/backward bending of the trunk produces a rotation of the pelvic girdle on top of the femoral heads. A full, symmetrical squat may be difficult to achieve when femoral flexion is limited. If the articular and myofascial structures posterior to the hip joint are tight, anterior displacement of the femoral head can occur leading to impingement of the labrum, capsule and possibly the iliopsoas bursa and tendon (groin pain) during this maneuver (Ratzlaff, personal communication). Lateral bending of the trunk will be restricted such that the pelvic girdle cannot translate in the coronal plane without deviation when abduction or adduction is limited.

The hypomobile hip has little effect on the ipsilateral rotation tests (both posterior and anterior) except that the sacroiliac joint motion begins earlier in the range. The supine and prone active straight leg raise tests are performed without difficulty and minimal restrictions may not be evident during these tests.

Articular mobility/stability tests

The osteokinematic tests of physiological mobility at the hip disclose the pattern of restriction which can be either articular or myofascial. The fully established capsular pattern of restriction (Cyriax 1954) of the hip joint is:

1. 50°–55° limitation of femoral abduction
2. 0° of femoral medial rotation from neutral
3. 90° limitation of femoral flexion
4. 10°–30° limitation of femoral extension
5. femoral lateral rotation and adduction is fully maintained.

However, as was previously mentioned, the degenerative process of the hip joint occurs over time such that, in the presence of early pathology, the only objective finding may be a slight limitation of medial rotation and flexion. As the pathology progresses, the full capsular pattern of restriction emerges.

The quadrant test is universally affected when the joint is hypomobile (Grieve 1983). Often, a painful 'bump' can be palpated during the flexion/adduction phase of the test, associated with muscular resistance (hypertonicity) and reactive spasm if the joint is irritable. Recently, this has been thought (Ratzlaff, personal communication) to be the result of impingement of the anterior structures of the hip when the posterior articular and myofascial structures become tight.

The end feel of motion during mobility testing can differentiate the articular restriction from the myofascial. A very hard end feel is indicative of an articular restriction whereas a softer end feel is usually muscular. Clinically, the two are usually seen in combination given the intimate articular neuromuscular physiology.

The tests for articular stability are normal when the hip is hypomobile. Proprioception and *dynamic* stability, however, are often deficient due to the altered neurophysiology.

Muscle function tests

Janda (1978, 1986) has observed that very early in the degenerative process of the hip joint, certain muscle groups respond by tightening while others respond by becoming weak. This muscle imbalance contributes to abnormal movement patterns and ultimately the lumbar spine, pelvic girdle and/or hip decompensates.

The muscles relative to the hip which tend to tighten include the hamstrings, rectus femoris, iliopsoas, tensor fascia lata, adductors and piriformis.

The muscles which tend to weaken include the gluteus maximus, medius and minimus. The effect of sustained muscle imbalance of the hip has been noted to enhance degenerative changes in the lumbar spine.

The inhibitory effect of a tight postural muscle is evidenced when weakness of the gluteus maximus accompanies tightness of the iliopsoas. Hip extension is slightly abnormal, lumbar lordosis tends to increase and abnormal loading of the lumbo-sacral segment initiates chronic changes which can be a cause of pain, in both low back and hip (Grieve 1983).

Sign of the buttock

According to Cyriax (1954), all major lesions or serious pathology in the buttock present with

…an arresting pattern of physical signs that draws immediate attention to the buttock. Passive hip flexion with the knee held extended … is slightly limited and painful. Passive hip flexion, this time with the knee flexed too, is again limited and more painful. Further examination reveals a non-capsular pattern of limitation of movement at the hip joint.

The end feel of motion is empty (i.e. limited by pain) as opposed to that of articular or myofascial tissue resistance.

This sign should alert the examiner to the potential presence of serious pathology such as:

1. osteomyelitis of the upper femur
2. chronic septic sacroiliac arthritis
3. ischiorectal abscess
4. septic bursitis
5. rheumatic fever with bursitis
6. neoplasm at the upper femur
7. iliac neoplasm
8. fractured sacrum.

If the 'sign of the buttock' is manifested during the examination, the presence/absence of serious pathology should be confirmed prior to initiating treatment.

Treatment of the hypomobile hip joint

Treatment of the hip joint forms part of the overall rehabilitation of the lumbo-pelvic-hip complex. To review, the ultimate goal is to restore the ability to control and transfer load from the trunk to the lower extremity. The following section outlines the specific therapy indicated during each stage of repair (i.e. substrate, fibroblastic, maturation) when localized hypomobility of the hip joint is found.

Substrate phase

During the first 4 to 6 days after injury, the goal of treatment is hemostasis of the wound. At home, the frequent application of ice together with rest is the treatment of choice.

At the clinic, electrotherapeutic analgesic modalities such as transcutaneous nerve stimulation and interferential current therapy can afford relief from pain; however, the patient should not attend at this stage if the physical stresses induced are greater than the relief gained.

Fibroblastic phase

With the resolution of active range of movement, the osteokinematic restriction becomes apparent. If the pattern of restriction is capsular, the joint is implicated as the etiological factor. If the pattern of restriction is non-capsular, the extra-articular tissues are implicated as the etiological factor. With respect to the articular tissues, the goal of treatment during this stage of repair is primarily to restore mobility. Passive mobilization techniques are utilized to restore the articular kinematics, combined with a specific home exercise program.

Lateral translation: passive mobilization technique (Fig. 10.1). This is a useful preliminary mobilization technique which can be graded

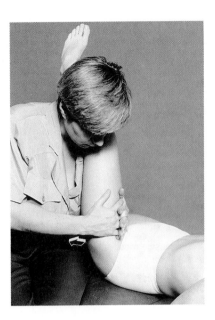

Figure 10.1 Passive mobilization of the hip joint: lateral translation.

according to the irritability of the joint. Initially, gentle grades are indicated, keeping well within the range of pain and reactive muscle spasm. The large afferent fiber input from the mechanoreceptors located in the articular capsule inhibits the centripetal transmission of the small fiber input (nociception) at the spinal cord, thus reducing the perception of pain via the spinal gating mechanism (see Ch. 4).

With the patient lying supine, the proximal thigh is palpated while the distal leg rests over the therapist's shoulder. The joint is distracted by applying a distolateral force parallel to the neck of the femur. The posteroanterior orientation of the applied force will vary and depends on the degree of femoral anteversion present.

Distraction: passive mobilization technique (Fig. 10.2). With the patient lying supine, the proximal thigh is palpated. The superior aspect of the hip joint is distracted by applying an inferolateral force along the longitudinal axis of the femur. This technique is also graded in accordance with the irritability of the joint. The neurophysiological effects have been described above.

Anteroposterior glide: passive mobilization technique (Fig. 10.3). With the patient lying

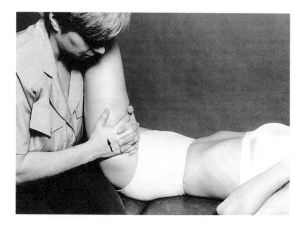

Figure 10.2   Passive mobilization of the hip joint: distraction.

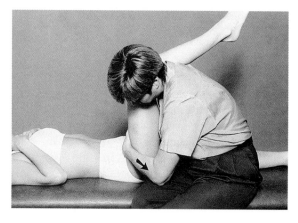

Figure 10.3   Passive mobilization of the hip joint: anteroposterior glide.

supine, the proximal thigh is palpated. An anteroposterior glide is induced by applying a posterolateral force parallel to the plane of the acetabular fossa. The technique is graded according to the level of joint irritability.

The restoration of optimal femoral function ultimately requires attention to both the articular and the myofascial system.

Home exercise program. Range of motion exercises which are directed towards resolving the individual's specific pattern of restriction are indicated at this stage of repair. If unilateral weight bearing is still painful, all weight-bearing exercises should be avoided.

Maturation phase

Mobilization techniques. If restrictive capsular adhesions have developed during the fibroblastic stage of repair, stronger passive mobilization techniques will be required to restore the optimal kinematic function of the hip joint. The passive mobilization techniques for this stage of repair are identical to those previously described except that the joint is taken strongly and specifically to the physiological limit of range (Grade 4).

NORMAL MOBILITY WITH PAIN

The presence of normal mobility at the hip joint associated with pain may be indicative of:

1. a mild inflammatory intra-articular process secondary to trauma, and/or overuse of the articular and myofascial tissues in compensation for altered function elsewhere;
2. an isolated ligament sprain following an athletic injury and/or other major trauma;
3. a muscle sprain following an athletic injury and/or other major trauma;
4. an inflamed bursa (iliopsoas, gluteal, ischial, trochanteric).

Traumatic arthritis

A mild inflammatory intra-articular process (mild traumatic arthritis) is painful but does not restrict the range of motion at the hip joint. Although walking aggravates the symptoms, the gait pattern is within normal limits. The specific mobility tests which reproduce the pain are consistent with those that are restricted in the capsular pattern (i.e. medial rotation and flexion). Compression of the joint is painful whereas distraction affords relief.

In the absence of any known trauma, the etiology of decompensation may lie extrinsic to the hip joint itself.

Ligament sprains

Isolated ligament sprains of this joint are rare in clinical practice. The major ligaments about the hip joint are among the strongest in the body and a fracture will usually occur before the ligament is sprained. Rarely, an isolated ligament injury occurs in combination with a myofascial sprain following a major traumatic incident which rapidly takes the joint beyond its normal range. The sports in which such injuries can occur are those which demand excessive articular mobility including gymnastics, dancing and the martial arts, as well as those in which excessive trauma is easily encountered such as soccer, skiing, football and ice skating.

The location of pain is usually specific to the damaged tissue and aggravated by motions which stress the injured tissue. If the hip joint is restricted by the lesion, the pattern of restriction is non-capsular. In the acute injury, resisted muscle tests may also be painful if the muscle being tested pulls on the lesioned ligament.

Muscle sprains

Contractile tissue lesions (i.e. muscle sprains) about the hip are commonly seen in athletes. The degree of injury is dependent upon the extent of trauma encountered. The mode of onset is definitely traumatic and the individual usually reports a 'snapping' sensation at the time of injury. If the injury is major, a tense hematoma rapidly develops at the wound site. In minor injuries, the onset may be insidious over a longer period of time and is not necessarily accompanied by a hematoma. The pain is localized to the damaged tissue and aggravated by movements which stress the lesioned tissue. The pattern of restriction, if any, is non-capsular.

The resisted muscle tests are consistently painful when the lesioned tissue is recruited. The muscles commonly injured include the rectus femoris, the hamstrings and the adductor muscles.

Bursitis

Bursitis about the hip joint is not rare. Acute bursitis is extremely painful, with most motions of the joint being restricted by pain as opposed to muscle or capsular tissue (i.e. the end feel is empty). The resisted muscle tests can also reproduce pain if the contraction compresses an inflamed bursa. Treatment requires a complete evaluation of the biomechanics of the lumbo-pelvic-hip complex and all articular and myofasical dysfunction must be addressed.

11

Muscles, posture and ergonomics

The successful rehabilitation of the lumbo-pelvic-hip complex requires the restoration of efficient myofascial and postural function. In addition, the employment of optimal static and dynamic ergonomics (i.e. sitting and standing postures, walking and lifting biomechanics) is essential if a recurrence is to be prevented. Following the restoration of articular function within the lumbo-pelvic-hip complex, attention should be directed towards the muscles which have either tightened and/or weakened, since the abnormal movement patterns they produce may persist long after the articular function has been restored. Sahrmann's (White & Sahrmann 1994) muscle system balance theory suggests that there is an ideal resting length for each muscle. When muscle strength is tested in this ideal position, the muscle will be strong. A muscle which habitually functions in a lengthened position will increase its number of sarcomeres whereas a muscle functioning in a shortened position will lose sarcomeres (Williams & Goldspink 1978). In either case, the muscle will test weak when resisted in a neutral joint position since this is no longer the ideal position. Treatment must address the restoration of optimal muscle length.

STRETCHING FOR MUSCLES WHICH TEND TO TIGHTEN

The muscles which tend to tighten/shorten include the erector spinae, quadratus lumborum, hamstrings, rectus femoris, iliopsoas, tensor fascia lata, adductors, piriformis and the deep

153

external rotators of the hip. Clinically, the tight muscles produce a restriction or deviation of motion in the functional tests (Ch. 7) *in the presence of normal articular mobility*. The treatment includes active mobilization techniques combined with a specific home exercise program designed to restore the optimal length of the muscle.

Erector spinae and quadratus lumborum

Active mobilization technique (Fig. 11.1)

With the patient sitting, feet supported, arms crossed and the vertebral column in a neutral position, the contralateral shoulder is palpated with the ventral arm. The ipsilateral erector spinae/quadratus lumborum muscle group is stretched by laterally bending the patient away from and rotating the patient towards the therapist to the limit of the physiological range of motion. The myofascia on the side of the produced convexity should now be on stretch.

The patient is instructed to hold this position while the therapist attempts to further increase the lateral bend/rotation components of the stretch. The isometric contraction is held for up to 5 seconds followed by a period of complete relaxation. The thoracolumbar spine is taken to the new limit of lateral bend/rotation and the technique repeated from this point.

Home exercise (Fig. 11.2)

The patient is instructed to start from the four-point kneeling position, and to flex the thoracolumbar spine by kyphosing in a posterior direction. While maintaining this kyphosis, the patient sits back on the heels, without displacing the hands, until an initial stretch of the spinal extensors is perceived. At no time should the stretch produce pain since this would result in a muscle contraction and defeat the purpose of the stretch (Stark 1997). This position is maintained until the sensation of tension has passed (30 seconds to 1 minute) and is followed by an increase in the sit back. After the tension has been released a second time the patient returns to the four-point kneeling position. The stretch is repeated as often as possible during the day.

Hamstrings

Active mobilization (Fig. 11.3)

With the patient lying supine, the lower extremity is palpated above the ankle. While

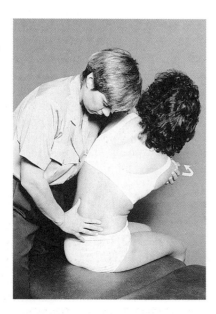

Figure 11.1 Active mobilization technique for the left erector spinae and quadratus lumborum muscles.

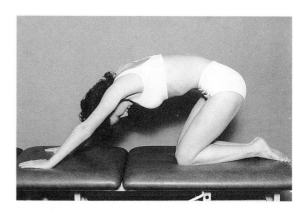

Figure 11.2 Home exercise for stretching the spinal extensor muscles.

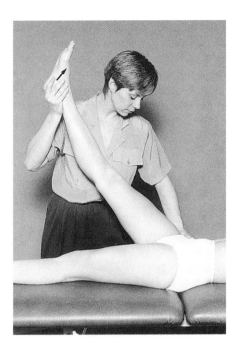

Figure 11.3 Active mobilization technique for the hamstring muscles.

maintaining the knee in extension, the femur is flexed at the hip joint. The therapist's cranial hand monitors any subsequent posterior rotation of the innominate via the anterior aspect of the iliac crest and the anterior superior iliac spine (ASIS). The extensibility of the hamstring muscle group has been reached when the innominate is felt to posteriorly rotate.

The patient is instructed to hold this position while the therapist attempts to increase the femoral flexion at the hip joint. The most effective contraction for this technique is usually isometric and is held for up to 5 seconds followed by a period of complete relaxation. The femur is taken to the new limit of flexion and the technique is repeated from this point.

To specifically stretch the individual muscles of the hamstring muscle group, the starting position of the femur and the tibia may be altered in the following manner: biceps femoris — medially rotate/adduct the femur and medially rotate the tibia; semimembranosus/ semitendinosus — laterally rotate/abduct the femur and laterally rotate the tibia.

Home exercise (Fig. 11.4)

With the patient supine, the femur is flexed at the hip joint to 90° and the foot is supported against a wall. The foot is slowly slid up the wall thus extending the knee until the first tension is perceived within the hamstring muscle belly (not the tendon insertion or origin) (Stark 1997). At no time should the stretch produce pain since this would result in a muscle contraction and defeat the purpose of the stretch (Stark 1997). This position is maintained until the sensation of tension has passed (30 seconds to 1 minute) and is followed by an increase in extension of the knee. The stretch is repeated twice during each session and several sessions are required each day.

The exercise can be modified to specifically stretch the medial or lateral hamstring by altering the starting position of the lower extremity. Medial rotation of the femur combined with slight adduction will maximally stretch the biceps femoris muscle. Lateral rotation of the femur combined with slight abduction will maximally stretch the semimembranosus and semitendinosus muscles.

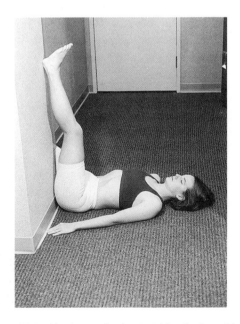

Figure 11.4 Home exercise for stretching the hamstring muscles.

Iliopsoas

Active mobilization (Fig. 11.5)

With the patient supine, lying at the end of the table, one femur is flexed while maintaining a neutral lumbar spine. This knee is held by the patient and the foot is supported against the therapist's lateral thorax. The anterior aspect of the iliac crest and the ASIS of the limb being stretched are palpated with the cranial hand. With the caudal hand, the femur is guided into extension, supporting the extended knee, until the physiological length of the iliopsoas muscle has been reached.

The patient is instructed to hold this position while the therapist releases support of the femur. The isometric contraction is held for up to 5 seconds followed by a period of complete relaxation. The femur is taken to the new limit of extension and the technique repeated from this point.

Maximal stretching of the iliopsoas muscle (Fig. 11.6) is achieved by having the patient lie prone, with the vertebral column laterally flexed away from the muscle being stretched and the non-involved extremity supported on the floor such that the femur is flexed at the hip joint (Evjenth & Hamberg 1984a,b). The involved extremity is then medially rotated at the hip joint with the knee flexed to 90° and supported in this position by the therapist. Femoral extension is achieved by elevating the end of the table. The active mobilization is performed by instructing the patient to flex the femur into the table, to hold the contraction for up to 5 seconds and then to completely relax. The femur is passively taken to the new physiological range of motion and the mobilization repeated.

Home exercise

This muscle is very difficult to effectively stretch without assistance. The best method is to teach a partner the active mobilization procedure. According to Stark (1997), exercises which aim to lengthen a muscle in a weight-bearing position are ineffective since the muscle is contracting to assist in stabilization. Stretching in this way puts more tension on the muscle/tendon or tendon/bone junction. Stark feels that this can lead to breakdown of the musculotendinous and/or tenoperiosteal junction both of which are not anatomically designed to stretch. If the goal is to restore the optimal resting length of the

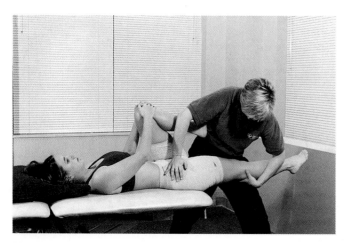

Figure 11.5

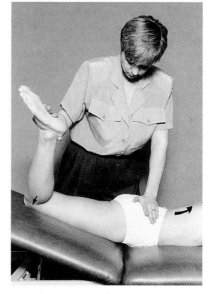

Figure 11.6

Figures 11.5 and 11.6 Two active mobilization techniques for the iliopsoas muscle.

muscle, all stretches should be completely passive.

Rectus femoris

Active mobilization (Fig. 11.7)

With the patient supine, lying at the end of the table, one femur is flexed while maintaining a neutral lumbar spine. This knee is held by the patient and the foot is supported against the therapist's lateral thorax. The anterior aspect of the iliac crest and the ASIS of the limb being stretched are palpated with the cranial hand. With the caudal hand, the femur is guided into extension, with the knee flexed, until the physiological length of the rectus femoris muscle has been reached.

The patient is instructed to hold this position while the therapist attempts to flex the knee further. The isometric contraction is held for up to 5 seconds followed by a period of complete relaxation. The tibia is taken to the new limit of flexion and the technique repeated from this point.

Maximal stretching of the rectus femoris muscle (Fig. 11.8) is achieved by having the patient lie prone with the non-involved extremity supported on the floor such that the femur is flexed at the hip joint (Evjenth & Hamberg 1984a,b). The involved extremity is then flexed at the knee joint to the physiological limit and supported in this position by the therapist. Further stretch is achieved by extending the femur at the hip joint by elevating the end of the table. The active mobilization is performed by instructing the patient to flex the femur into the table and to extend the tibia against the therapist's resistance. The contraction is held for up to 5 seconds followed by a period of complete relaxation. The tibia and the femur are passively taken to the new physiological range of motion and the mobilization repeated.

Home exercise (Fig. 11.9)

With the patient standing or side-lying (Stark 1997), the femur is initially flexed at the hip joint and the tibia flexed at the knee joint. The ankle is grasped just proximal to the talocrural joint and the knee flexion maintained while the femur is passively extended at the hip joint until first tension is perceived in the rectus femoris muscle (not at the tendinous junctions). This position is maintained until the sensation of tension has passed (30 seconds to 1 minute) and is followed by an increase in extension of the hip. The stretch

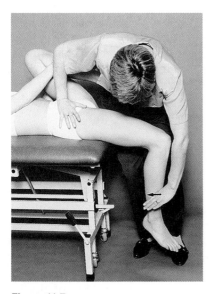

Figure 11.7

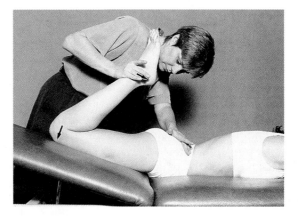

Figure 11.8

Figures 11.7 and 11.8   Two active mobilization techniques for the rectus femoris muscle.

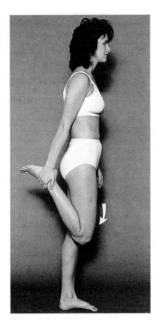

Figure 11.9 Home exercise for stretching the rectus femoris muscle.

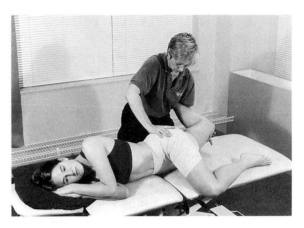

Figure 11.10 Active mobilization technique for the tensor fascia lata muscle.

is repeated twice during each session and several sessions are required each day.

Tensor fascia lata

Active mobilization (Fig. 11.10)

To actively mobilize the right tensor fascia lata muscle, the patient is positioned in right side-lying with the left hip and knee comfortably flexed. The anterolateral aspect of the right femur is grasped with the caudal hand and the flexed right knee supported by the therapist's caudal hand and forearm. The cranial hand stabilizes the posterior aspect of the pelvic girdle. The femur is taken to the physiological limit of the tensor fascia lata muscle by passively extending, adducting and laterally rotating the femur at the hip joint.

From this position, the patient is instructed to resist further extension, adduction and lateral rotation of the femur. The isometric contraction is held for up to 5 seconds followed by a period of complete relaxation. The femur is taken to the new limit of extension, adduction and lateral

rotation and the technique repeated from this point.

Home exercise

According to Stark (1997), this muscle should not be stretched in any weight-bearing position since this posture requires it to contract for stabilization of the pelvic girdle. The anterior band of the tensor fascia lata muscle is often short and dominant when the posterior gluteal muscles (maximus, medius and minimus) are lengthened and weak. The resting length of this muscle can be restored by increasing the strength of the posterior gluteal group (see below). If further length is required from the tensor fascia lata, it is best achieved with manual assistance (active mobilization techniques).

Adductors

Active mobilization (Fig. 11.11)

With the patient supine, lying at the end of the table, one femur is flexed while maintaining a neutral lumbar spine. This knee is held by the patient and the foot is supported against the therapist's lateral thorax. The anterior aspect of the iliac crest and the ASIS of the limb being stretched are palpated with the cranial hand. With the caudal hand, the femur is guided into

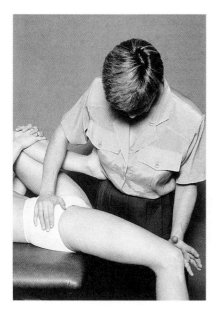

Figure 11.11 Active mobilization technique for the adductor muscles.

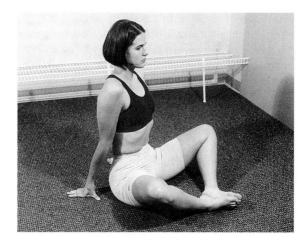

Figure 11.12 Home exercise for stretching the adductor muscles.

abduction until the physiological limit of the adductor muscles has been reached. The degree of femoral flexion/extension, medial/lateral rotation can be varied according to the pattern of restriction found.

The patient is instructed to resist further abduction from this position. The isometric contraction is held for up to 5 seconds followed by a period of complete relaxation. The femur is taken to the new limit of abduction and the technique repeated from this point.

Home exercise (Fig. 11.12)

With the patient sitting, back supported, the femurs are abducted and laterally rotated such that the soles of the feet are approximated. The knees are slowly allowed to drop towards the floor until first tension is perceived in the adductor muscle bellies (not at the tendinous junctions). This position is maintained until the sensation of tension has passed (30 seconds to 1 minute) and is followed by an increase in abduction/lateral rotation of the hip. The stretch is repeated twice during each session and several sessions are required each day.

Piriformis and the deep external rotators of the hip

Active mobilization (Fig. 11.13)

With the patient lying supine, the lower extremity is grasped at the flexed knee. The lateral aspect of the iliac crest and the ASIS are palpated with the cranial hand while the caudal

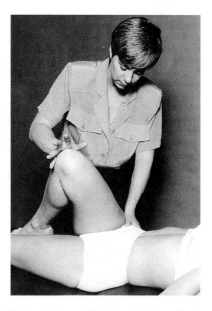

Figure 11.13 Active mobilization technique for the piriformis muscle.

hand flexes the femur to 60° of flexion. At this point, the piriformis muscle acts as a pure abductor of the femur. Before 60° it also laterally rotates the femur, while after 60° it medially rotates the femur. From 60° of femoral flexion, the femur is guided into adduction with the caudal hand while the cranial hand monitors the subsequent medial rotation of the innominate. The maximal extensibility of the piriformis muscle has been reached when the innominate is felt to medially rotate, and although further adduction of the femur is possible, it is secondary to the medial rotation of the innominate. If the femur is taken beyond 60° of flexion, lateral femoral rotation is also required to fully stretch the muscle.

The patient is instructed to resist further adduction from this position (if the femur is flexed to 60°), to resist adduction/lateral rotation (if the femur is flexed beyond 60°), and adduction/medial rotation (if the femur is flexed less than 60°). The isometric contraction is held for up to 5 seconds followed by a period of complete relaxation. The femur   is taken to the new limit of adduction/rotation and the technique repeated from this point.

Home exercise (Fig. 11.14)

To stretch the right posterior external rotators, the patient lies supine and the right femur is flexed and laterally rotated such that the right ankle rests on the flexed left knee. The patient grasps the posterior aspect of the distal left thigh. From this position, the left hip is flexed until first tension is perceived in the right buttock. This position is maintained until the sensation of tension has passed (30 seconds to 1 minute) and is followed by an increase in flexion of the left hip. The stretch is repeated twice during each session and several sessions are required each day.

AN EXERCISE PROGRAM FOR STABILIZATION

When the lumbar spine and/or pelvic girdle are unable to transfer load efficiently, rehabilitation must address the strength, endurance and

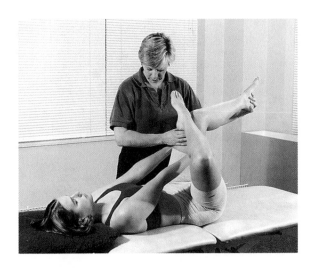

Figure 11.14   Home exercise for stretching the piriformis muscle and the deep external rotators of the hip.

timing of recruitment of the inner and outer unit of muscles (Chs 5, 7). The aim of this program is to isolate the appropriate muscles, retrain their holding capacity, and their ability to automatically contract appropriately with other synergists to support and protect the spine/pelvic girdle under various functional loads (Lee 1997b). Richardson & Jull (1994, 1995) and more recently, Richardson, Jull, Hodges & Hides (1997) have devised a four-stage program designed primarily to isolate and train the inner unit (Table 11.1). They feel that slow controlled movements with increasing loads is what most people need to restore function. The principles of this program are outlined in Table 11.2.

The exercises should be performed slowly with tonic contractions encouraged over phasic ones. No fast ballistic movements are allowed. Exercises which facilitate co-contraction of muscle groups are encouraged as opposed to unidirectional exercises. The focus is on control of the neutral joint position under low loads. When the principles of this program are subsequently applied to the activation of the outer unit (Vleeming et al 1995b, 1997) a very effective rehabilitation program can be achieved.

The first stage of the program (stage 1) requires isolation of the muscles of the inner unit (transversus abdominis, multifidus and the

Table 11.1 Stabilization program (Richardson, Jull, Hodges & Hides 1997)

Stage 1
Isolate the muscles of the inner unit
Train the muscles of the inner unit

Stage 2
Isolate the muscles of the outer unit while maintaining inner unit control
Isolate individual muscles of the outer unit systems as necessary
Decrease the base of support and increase the load

Stage 3
Control motions through the lumbar spine and pelvic girdle while maintaining inner unit control

Stage 4
Maintain stabilization with high speed motions

Table 11.2 Principles of stabilization training (Richardson, Jull, Hodges & Hides 1997)

- Exercises should facilitate tonic *not* phasic contractions

- No fast ballistic movements are allowed

- Exercises should involve co-contraction and not be unidirectional

- Focus on neutral joint position and low load initially

- Progress by maintaining trunk position and increasing load in more unstable environments

pelvic floor). Once the patient can effectively isolate this unit, it is trained by requiring 10 repetitions of 10-second holds. This will help to build endurance.

The second stage of the program (stage 2) requires activation of the outer unit (posterior oblique, anterior oblique, deep longitudinal or lateral systems) while maintaining a holding contraction of the inner unit. This is achieved by introducing limb movement, reducing the base of support and then increasing the load.

Stage 3 involves stabilization during controlled movement of the lumbar spine and pelvic girdle and stage 4 requires stabilization during high-speed motions. Very few people require stage 4 stabilization. In fact, high-speed exercise has been shown (Richardson & Jull 1995) to reduce the ability to stabilize the trunk.

Isolation and training of the inner unit

Pelvic floor: levator ani

The exercise instruction begins with teaching the patient the location of this muscle. Following this, they are instructed to shorten the distance between the coccyx and the pubic symphysis. For women, a prompt to lift the pelvic floor, or their vagina, internally (Kegel exercise) can facilitate the understanding of the exercise.

When the muscle contracts properly, the transversus abdominis can be felt to co-contract at a point 2 cm medial and inferior to the ASIS. This is a useful point of palpation for both the therapist and patient to ensure the exercise is being done correctly. In addition, the therapist can palpate the sacral apex posteriorly. When the levator ani contracts, the sacrum will counter-nutate relative to the innominates with no motion occurring between the pelvic girdle and the lumbar spine or the pelvic girdle and the legs. The patient is instructed to hold the contraction for 10 seconds and to repeat the exercise 10 times.

Often, they will try to substitute with other muscles. When gluteus maximus is used, the pelvis will posteriorly tilt and the buttocks can be felt to contract. This is a common substitution strategy. When done properly, the buttock is relaxed and no movement of the pelvic girdle occurs.

Transversus abdominis/multifidus

These muscles are isolated in the same manner as they are tested (see Ch. 7) (Richardson & Jull 1995, Richardson et al 1997) (Figs 7.49, 7.50). The holding capacity is trained by asking the patient to perform their maximum number of 10-second holds. It is useful to monitor transversus abdominis activation at the palpation point noted above (2 cm medial and inferior to the ASIS). This will ensure that the appropriate contraction is occurring during all repetitions. The multifidus can be monitored lateral to the spinous processes of the lumbar spine. When the inner unit fatigues, the outer unit (external/internal oblique, erector spinae) will take over.

The training is progressed from the four-point kneeling position to sitting and then to standing. The number of repetitions may vary between exercise sessions depending on the level of fatigue. The goal is to reach 10 repetitions of 10-second holds.

Isolation and training of the outer unit

The stabilization program is progressed to stage 2 by introducing lower or upper extremity motion (outer unit activation and control) while controlling the inner unit. There are many ways this can be achieved and the examples which follow are merely suggestions.

In the supine position with the hips and knees flexed, the patient is required to isolate the inner unit, maintain the lumbar neutral position (some recruitment of the anterior and posterior oblique systems will be required) and to slowly let the knee fall to one side (Fig. 11.15). Alternatively, they may extend the leg with the foot supported on the table (a slippery surface is helpful during the initial stages of this exercise) (Fig. 11.16).

The load may be increased in this same position, by asking the patient to lift the foot off the table while maintaining the hip and knee

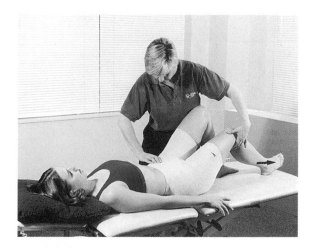

Figure 11.16 One leg extension with support with co-contraction of the inner unit; stage 2.

flexed. A further progression would be to slowly extend this leg (with the foot lifted) to 45° above the table (Fig. 11.17). This is initially performed unilaterally and can be progressed to alternate leg extensions. The same exercises may be performed sitting on a gym ball or lying supine on a long roll. By making the base unstable, the exercise becomes more difficult without moving into the next stage.

Exercise rolls and gym balls facilitate the automatic reactions necessary for function (Farrell et al 1994, Irion 1992). Exercising on a

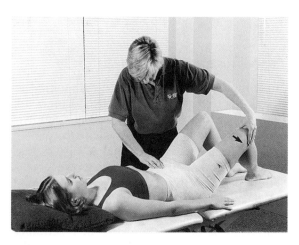

Figure 11.15 Bent knee fall out with co-contraction of the inner unit; stage 2.

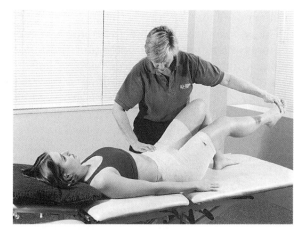

Figure 11.17 One leg extension supine with co-contraction of the inner unit; stage 2.

gym ball requires core stability (inner unit control), coordination and appropriate reflexes. While sitting on the ball, the patient is instructed to contract the pelvic floor, transversus abdominis and multifidus, or in other words, to contract the inner unit. They are then instructed to maintain this contraction and move forwards and back, and up and down on the ball (Fig. 11.18). The same exercise can be done in standing with weight shifting from side to side, forward and back. At home, the patient is instructed to incorporate the co-contraction of the inner unit into their activities of daily living. Figures 11.19–11.23 illustrate the way the principles of core stability can be incorporated into an exercise program at this stage, with variety and challenge.

If the individual muscles of an outer unit system are weak or poorly recruited, the exercise program should include isolation and training at this time. In the posterior oblique system, it is common to find the gluteus maximus both

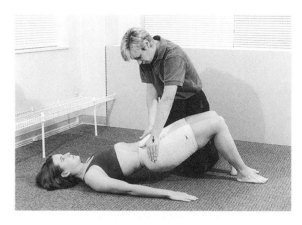

Figure 11.19 Bridge and resist trunk rotation (therapist applies resistance through the pelvic girdle); stage 2.

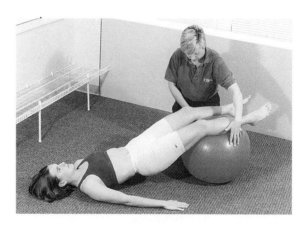

Figure 11.20 Bridge and resist motion of lower extremities (force is applied to gym ball by the therapist); stage 2.

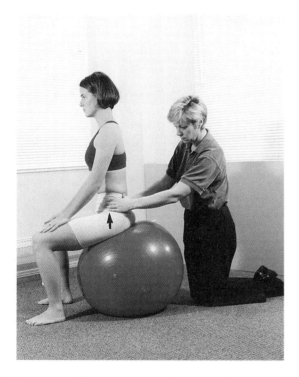

Figure 11.18 Rise and sit with co-contraction of the inner unit; stage 2.

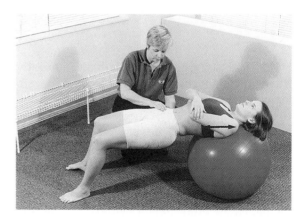

Figure 11.21 Bridge and roll forward and back with the gym ball supporting only the upper thorax, head and neck.

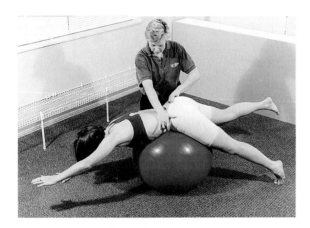

Figure 11.22 Prone over ball, one leg, one arm extension with co-contraction of the inner unit; stage 2.

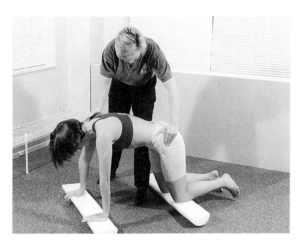

Figure 11.23 Four-point kneeling on two half-rolls; resistance can be applied by therapist to motion in many planes.

The lever arm is increased (and thus the load) by lifting the extended thigh.

Leg extension machines (Apex leg press, Medical Exercise Thigh Trainer, Shuttle MVP or 2000-1) can help to strengthen the gluteal group. On the Shuttle, the patient can initially exercise in the supine position with either one or two feet on the foot plate. With the trunk stabilized, they push against a variable resistance which can be increased as tolerated (Fig. 11.25). They are progressed from this position to four-point kneeling (more unstable base) (Fig. 11.26). This is still a stage 2 exercise.

Functional training can be introduced by having the patient practice going from sitting to

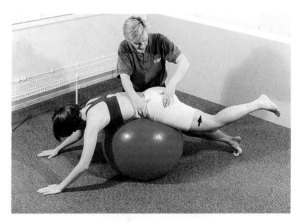

Figure 11.24 Isolation of gluteus maximus, prone over gym ball with co-contraction of the inner unit.

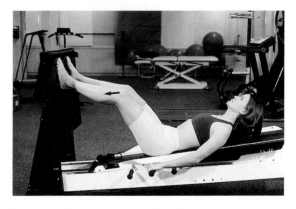

Figure 11.25 Strengthening of the leg extensors with co-contraction of the inner unit on a Shuttle MVP.

lengthened (secondary to a habitually anteriorly tilted pelvic girdle) and weak (due to lengthening and also secondary to inhibition from the sacroiliac joint). The gluteus maximus is isolated by having the patient squeeze the buttocks together and sustain the contraction for 10 seconds. A surface electromyography (EMG) unit can provide a useful biofeedback system for this muscle. The exercise is progressed by having the patient lie prone over a gym ball and asking them to initially recruit the inner unit and then extend the hip with the knee flexed (Fig. 11.24).

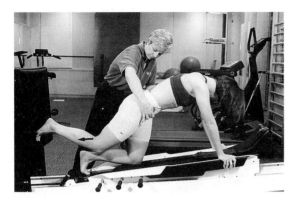

Figure 11.26 Strengthening of one leg extensor in four-point kneeling with a balance challenge on a Shuttle MVP.

standing with a stabilized trunk, using primarily the gluteus maximus (Fig. 11.27). To be done properly, this exercise requires control of the lumbar spine and pelvic girdle through the inner unit and a very strong buttock.

With respect to the lateral system, the posterior fibers of the gluteus medius are often weak. This can have profound effects on walking and load transference through the hip joint (Lee 1997a).

Commonly, the patient compensates for the weakness by adopting a Trendelenburg gait (Ch. 5). This gait can lead to decompensation of the soft tissues of the sacroiliac joint and the lumbar spine with symptoms ensuing.

Isolation of the gluteus medius is taught in the side-lying position with a pillow between the knees. The patient is shown where to palpate the muscle posteriorly and taught which compensatory movement strategies to avoid (rotation or sideflexion of the trunk). Initially, with or without a surface EMG unit, the patient is asked to lift the medial aspect of the knee off of the pillow (Fig. 11.28). Careful observation for substitution strategies is required at this stage. The exercise is progressed by asking the patient to lift the knee off of the pillow and then to extend the knee while maintaining the correct position of the trunk and hip. The knee is then flexed and lowered down onto the pillow. Resistance can be added using theraband or exercise machines such as the Shuttle. In addition, the Fitter can be used to rehabilitate the gluteus medius and the contralateral hip adductors while maintaining a stabilized trunk (Fig. 11.29).

Isolation of the anterior oblique system begins with training the specific contraction of the external and internal oblique abdominals. When the external obliques contract bilaterally, the

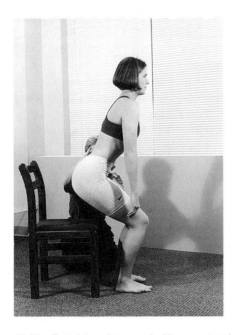

Figure 11.27 Retraining sit to stand with co-contraction of the inner unit.

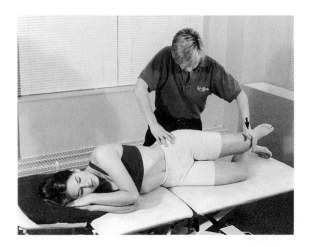

Figure 11.28 Isolation of the posterior fibers of gluteus medius.

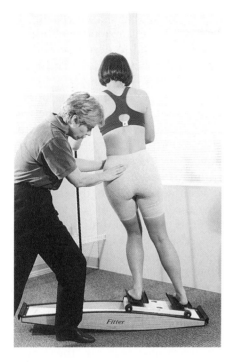

Figure 11.29 Strengthening of the lateral system with co-contraction of the inner unit on a Fitter.

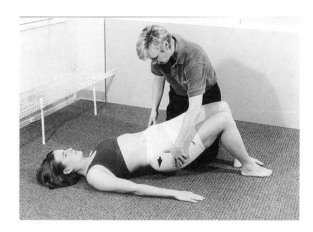

Figure 11.30 Bridge and rotate the trunk/pelvic girdle at the hip joints with co-contraction of the inner unit.

infrasternal angle narrows. When the internal obliques contract bilaterally, the infrasternal angle widens. The patient is taught to palpate the lateral costal margin and to specifically widen and narrow the infrasternal angle through specific contraction of the oblique abdominals. This is not a very functional exercise although it is important to be able to selectively recruit the four muscles of the abdominal wall.

The progression includes activation of the anterior and posterior oblique systems (maintaining inner unit control) and differentiation of trunk from femoral motion. To begin, the patient is supine with the hips and knees flexed. They are instructed to bridge and then to rotate the trunk/pelvic girdle at the hip joints in the unsupported position (Fig. 11.30). For this to remain a stage 2 exercise, the lumbar joints must stay in a neutral position.

To make this exercise functional, pulleys or theraband can be used. In a standing position, the patient is required to pull the weight down using a rotary motion, not through the trunk but through the hip joint (Fig. 11.31). This exercise requires effective stabilization of the trunk via the inner unit, active recruitment of the latissimus dorsi, gluteus maximus (posterior oblique system), gluteus medius (lateral system), contralateral adductors and the oblique abdominals (anterior oblique system). The load is increased as tolerated and the speed is maintained at a low level.

At this time, wobble boards or long rollers can be used to challenge balance in standing. The patient must stabilize the trunk and shift their weight from side to side, forward and back, do full squats or upper extremity work (Fig. 11.32). All exercise equipment can be used for stabilization therapy and only imagination limits the program once the principles are understood. Thus, exercises can be adapted to meet the demands of the patient's work and recreation. The program should be less 'muscle-specific' and more functionally oriented. It is important not to progress faster than the rate at which the motion/load can be controlled. The early stages are the most difficult to teach and often take the longest time to master, and diligence is rewarded with fewer setbacks. If limb motion is added, or the load is increased, beyond that which can be controlled by the inner unit, the pain will increase.

According to the protocol advocated by Richardson & Jull (1994), stage 3 exercises

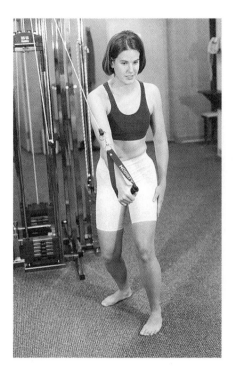

Figure 11.31   Rotation training using pulleys.

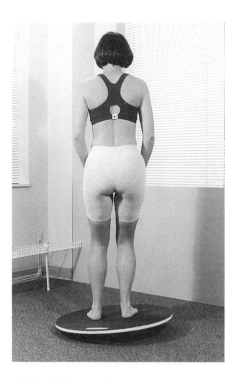

Figure 11.32   Balance challenge on a wobble board.

involve controlled motion *of the unstable region.* This stage is much more advanced and is only given when required by an individual's work or sport. Programs include concentric and eccentric work with variable resistance in all three planes, sagittal, coronal and transverse. At this stage, the various isokinetic machines (Medex, Medical exercise rotation trainer) as well as any pulley apparatus can be useful. Rotation is often not well tolerated by those with a true articular instability of the sacroiliac joint when the pelvis is fixed, either in an apparatus or in sitting. Before this exercise can be given, they must be able to stabilize the neutral zone with appropriate inner unit recruitment.

POSTURAL AND ERGONOMIC RETRAINING

Sitting

The ideal sitting position (Fig. 11.33) is one which maintains the spine in a neutral position,

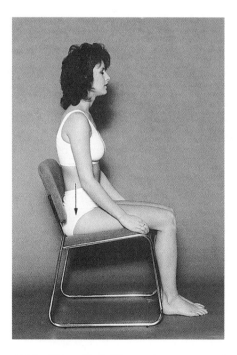

Figure 11.33   The optimal sitting posture preserves the natural cervical, thoracic and lumbar curves.

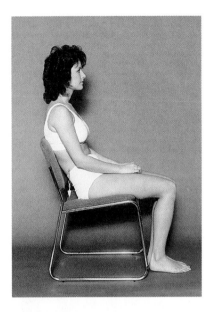 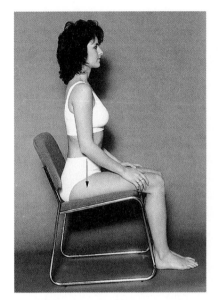

Figure 11.34   **Figure 11.35**

Figure 11.34 and 11.35   The 'slouched' and the 'over erect' sitting postures.

thus preserving the natural cervical, thoracic and lumbar curves, as well as directing the line of gravity through the lumbosacral junction along the arcuate lines of the innominates through to the ischial tuberosities. If the body weight is allowed to pass anterior or posterior to this ideal position (Figs 11.34, 11.35), excessive static stresses will be induced through the lumbo-pelvic-hip complex, thus facilitating breakdown of the tissues.

The average chair appears to be designed for the 5 ft 10 in (178 cm) man. Individuals less than this height must slide forward in the chair if the feet are to reach the ground. This motion places the line of gravity behind the ischial tuberosities, thus encouraging flexion of the lumbar vertebral column and the pelvic girdle (i.e. slouching). Individuals greater than this height have more difficulty controlling the optimal posture of the upper girdle. To reach a desk top, they must lower the trunk, thereby flexing the cervico-thoracic and thoracic portions of the vertebral column.

Adjusting the work height, as well as the visual field, is critical to successfully maintaining an optimal sitting posture. If the desk is too high, the shoulder girdle must be elevated to write, which can induce a lateral bend of the vertebral column. If the desk is too low, the shoulder girdle must descend, thus encouraging flexion of the vertebral column. Careful revision of the patient's sitting posture is required if the patient's occupation and/or leisure activity requires the habitual use of this position.

The goal is to position the lumbo-pelvic-hip complex in the optimal posture of balance such that the osseous components of the unit bear most of the stresses.

Standing

It has been shown (Basmajian & Deluca 1985) that among the mammals man has the most efficient posture in bipedal stance. In the lumbo-pelvic-hip region, intermittent bursts of activity from the gluteus medius, tensor fascia lata and hamstring muscles are required to control postural sway. Constant activity has been reported (Basmajian & Deluca 1985) in the iliopsoas muscle to support the iliofemoral ligament of the hip joint, as well as in the internal oblique muscle to protect the inguinal canal. All other muscle groups are quiescent when the standing posture is optimal. Deviation from this economical position results in the immediate recruitment of both the trunk and femoral musculature, thus dramatically increasing the energy expenditure of standing still.

Where is this optimal position? To review, if the body is viewed from the lateral aspect, a vertical line should pass through the following points (see Fig. 7.1):

1. the external auditory meatus
2. the bodies of the cervical vertebrae
3. the glenohumeral joint
4. slightly anterior to the bodies of the thoracic vertebrae transecting the vertebrae at the thoracolumbar junction
5. the bodies of the lumbar vertebrae
6. the sacral promontory
7. slightly posterior to the coronal axis of the hip joint
8. slightly anterior to the coronal axis of the knee joint
9. slightly anterior to the talocrural joint
10. the naviculocalcaneo-cuboid joint.

Fortunately, we are rarely required to stand perfectly still; however, some tasks, such as ironing, do require prolonged periods of relative immobility of the lower quadrant. If the position of optimal postural balance is lost, the energy expenditure required to stand still will increase. Excessive static stresses will then be placed on the tissues of the lumbo-pelvic-hip complex, facilitating their breakdown.

Frequently altering the standing posture is one means of coping with relative immobility. The habitual unilateral elevation of one foot onto a low stool should not be encouraged unless it is alternated with the opposite extremity. Ideally, the patient should be taught how to achieve the optimal posture of the lumbo-pelvic-hip complex as well as encouraged to frequently move both into and out of this position.

Lifting

The biomechanics of optimal lifting technique have been described in Chapter 5. If the myofascial function of the lumbo-pelvic-hip complex has been restored (see the beginning of this chapter), the patient should be able to learn to lift ideally. The key points to teach include the following.

1. Always recruit the inner unit prior to accepting any load through the vertebral column.
2. Avoid moving the load outside of the pedal base (i.e. keep the load close to the body). When transferring patients up/down the bed, the magnitude of the transfer must be confined to the coronal dimensions of the pedal base.
3. Test the weight of the load prior to actually lifting it, so that its weight is never assumed. Obviously, if the load is too heavy, help is required.

Optimal, and therefore safe, loading and unloading of the lumbo-pelvic-hip region can occur when the inner and outer unit muscle systems control the neutral zone of motion. The coordinated muscle response depends on complex peripheral and central feedback and feedforward mechanisms which integrate the osseous, articular and muscular function. Successful rehabilitation requires attention to all these aspects of the lumbo-pelvic-hip complex.

References

Abergel R P 1984 Biostimulation of procollagen production by low energy lasers in human skin fibroblast cultures. Journal of Investigative Dermatology 82: 395

Abitbol M M 1995 Energy storage in the vertebral column. In: Vleeming A, Mooney V, Dorman T, Snijders C (eds) Second interdisciplinary world congress on low back pain: the integrated function of the lumbar spine and sacroiliac joint, Part 1, San Diego, CA, 9–11 November, p 257

Abitbol M M 1997 Quadrupedalism, bipedalism, and human pregnancy. In: Vleeming A, Mooney V, Dorman T, Snijders C, Stoeckart R (eds) Movement, stability and low back pain. Churchill Livingstone, Edinburgh, ch 31, p 395

Adams M A, Dolan P 1997 The combined function of spine, pelvis, and legs when lifting with a straight back. In: Vleeming A, Mooney V, Dorman T, Snijders C, Stoeckart R (eds) Movement, stability and low back pain. Churchill Livingstone, Edinburgh, ch 14, p 195

Albee F H 1909 A study of the anatomy and the clinical importance of the sacroiliac joint. Journal of the American Medical Association 53: 1273

Astrom J 1975 Pre-operative effect of fenestration upon intraosseous pressures in patients with osteoarthrosis of the hip. Acta Orthopaedica Scandinavica 46: 963

Basmajian J V, Deluca C J 1985 Muscles alive: their functions revealed by electromyography. Williams & Wilkins, Baltimore

Bassett C A L 1968 Biologic significance of piezoelectricity. Calcified Tissue Research 1: 252

Beal M C 1982 The sacroiliac problem: review of anatomy, mechanics, and diagnosis. Journal of the American Osteopathic Association 81: 667

Bellamy N, Park W, Rooney P J 1983 What do we know about the sacroiliac joint? Seminars in Arthritis and Rheumatism 12: 282

Bogduk N L T 1983 The innervation of the lumbar spine. Spine 8: 286

Bogduk N L T 1997 Clinical anatomy of the lumbar spine and sacrum, 3rd edn. Churchill Livingstone, New York

Bowen V, Cassidy J D 1981 Macroscopic and microscopic anatomy of the sacroiliac joint from embryonic life until the eighth decade. Spine 6: 620

Bradlay K C 1985 The posterior primary rami of segmental nerves. In: Glasgow E F, Twomey, L T, Scull E R, Kleynhans A M (eds) Aspects of manipulative therapy, 2nd edn. Churchill Livingstone, Melbourne, ch 9, p 59

Brooke R 1924 The sacro-iliac joint. Journal of Anatomy 58: 299

Brooke R 1930 The pelvic joints during and after parturition and pregnancy. The Practitioner, London, p 307

Buyruk H M, Stam H J, Snijders C J, Vleeming A, Lameris J S, Holland W P J 1997 Measurement of sacroiliac joint stiffness with color Doppler imaging and the importance of asymmetric stiffness in sacroiliac pathology. In: Vleeming A, Mooney V, Dorman T, Snijders C, Stoeckart R (eds) Movement, stability and low back pain. Churchill Livingstone, Edinburgh, ch 24, p 297

Carmichael J P 1987 Inter- and intra-examiner reliability of palpation for sacroiliac joint dysfunction. Journal of Manipulative Physical Therapy 10(4): 164–171

Chamberlain W E 1930 The symphysis pubis in the roentgen examination of the sacroiliac joint. American Journal of Roentgenology 24: 621

Colachis S C, Worden R E, Bechtol C O, Strohm B R 1963 Movement of the sacroiliac joint in the adult male: a preliminary report. Archives of Physical Medicine and Rehabilitation 44: 490

Cooperman J M, Riddle D L, Rothstein J M 1990 Reliability and validity of judgments of the integrity of the anterior cruciate ligament of the knee using the Lachman's test. Physical Therapy 70(4): 225–233

Crock H V 1980 An atlas of the arterial supply of the head and neck of the femur in man. Clinical Orthopaedics and Related Research 152: 17

Cyriax J 1954 Textbook of orthopaedic medicine. Cassell, London

De Diemerbroeck I 1689 The anatomy of human bodies. Translated by W Salmon Brewster, London

Dee R 1969 Structure and function of hip joint innervation. Annals of the Royal College of Surgeons of England 45: 357

DonTigny R L 1985 Function and pathomechanics of the sacroiliac joint: a review. Physical Therapy 65: 35–44

DonTigny R L 1990 Anterior dysfunction of the sacroiliac joint as a major factor in the etiology of idiopathic low back pain syndrome. Physical Therapy 70: 250–265

DonTigny R L 1997 Mechanics and treatment of the sacroiliac joint. In: Vleeming A, Mooney V, Dorman T, Snijders C, Stoeckart R (eds) Movement, stability and low back pain. Churchill Livingstone, Edinburgh, ch 38, p 461

Dorman T 1994 Failure of self bracing at the sacroiliac joint: the slipping clutch syndrome. Journal of Orthopaedic Medicine 16: 49–51

Dorman T 1997 Pelvic mechanics and prolotherapy. In: Vleeming A, Mooney V, Dorman T, Snijders C, Stoeckart R (eds) Movement, stability and low back pain. Churchill Livingstone, Edinburgh, ch 40, p 501

Dreyfuss P, Dreyer S, Griffin J, Hoffman J, Walsh N 1994 Positive sacroiliac screening tests in asymptomatic adults. Spine 19: 1138–1143

Dreyfuss P, Michaelsen M, Pauza D, McLarty J, Bogduk N 1996 The value of history and physical examination in diagnosing sacroiliac joint pain. Spine 21: 2594–2602

Egund N, Olsson T H, Schmid H 1978 Movements in the sacro-iliac joints demonstrated with roentgen stereophotogrammetry. Acta Radiologica 19: 833

Encyclopedia Britannica 1981 15th edn, Vol 7. William Benter, Chicago

Evjenth O, Hamberg J 1984a Muscle stretching in manual therapy, a clinical manual; the spinal column and the

TM-joint. Alfta Rehab Forlag, Sweden

Evjenth O, Hamberg J 1984b Muscle stretching in manual therapy, a clinical manual; the extremities. Alfta Rehab Forlag, Sweden

Farfan H F 1973 Mechanical disorders of the low back. Lea & Febiger, Philadelphia

Farfan H F 1975 Muscular mechanism of the lumbar spine and the position of power and efficiency. Orthopedic Clinics of North America 8: 199

Farfan H F 1978 The biomechanical advantage of lordosis and hip extension for upright activity. Spine 3: 336

Farrell J, Drye C, Koury M 1994 Therapeutic exercise for back pain. In: Twomey L T, Taylor J R (eds) Physical therapy of the low back, 2nd edn. Churchill Livingstone, New York

Fortin J D, Dwyer A, West S, Pier J 1994a Sacroiliac joint pain referral patterns upon application of a new injection/arthrography technique. I: Asymptomatic volunteers. Spine 19(13): 1475–1482

Fortin J D, Dwyer A, Aprill C, Ponthieux B, Pier J 1994b Sacroiliac joint pain referral patterns. II: Clinical evaluation. Spine 19(13): 1483–1489

Fortin J D, Pier J, Falco F 1997 Sacroiliac joint injection: pain referral mapping and arthrographic findings. In: Vleeming A, Mooney V, Dorman T, Snijders C, Stoeckart R (eds) Movement, stability and low back pain. Churchill Livingstone, Edinburgh, ch 22, p 271

Fothergill W E 1896 Walcher's position in parturition. British Medical Journal 2: 1292

Fryette H H 1954 Principles of osteopathic technique. American Academy of Osteopathy, Colorado

Gandevia S C 1992 Some central and peripheral factors affecting human motorneuronal output in neuromuscular fatigue. Sports Medicine 13(2): 93–98

Gillies J H, Griesdale D E G 1997 The mystery of low-back pain. Canadian Journal of the Canadian Medical Education 9(9): 55–68

Gilmore K L 1986 Biomechanics of the lumbar motion segment. In: Grieve G P (ed) Modern manual therapy of the vertebral column. Churchill Livingstone, Edinburgh, ch 9, p 103

Goldthwait J E, Osgood R B 1905 A consideration of the pelvic articulations from an anatomical, pathological and clinical standpoint. Boston Medical and Surgical Journal 152: 593

Goodall J 1979 Life and death at Gombe. National Geographic 155(5): 592

Gracovetsky S 1997 Linking the spinal engine with the legs: a theory of human gait. In: Vleeming A, Mooney V, Dorman T, Snijders C, Stoeckart R (eds) Movement, stability and low back pain. Churchill Livingstone, Edinburgh, ch 20, p 243

Gracovetsky S, Farfan H F 1986 The optimum spine. Spine 11: 543

Gracovetsky S, Farfan H F, Lamy C 1981 The mechanism of the lumbar spine. Spine 6: 249

Gracovetsky S, Farfan H, Helluer C 1985 The abdominal mechanism. Spine 10: 317

Greenman P E 1990 Clinical aspects of sacroiliac function in walking. Journal of Manual Medicine 5: 125–130

Greenman P E 1990 Clinical aspects of the sacroiliac joint in walking. In: Vleeming A, Mooney V, Dorman T, Snijders C, Stoeckart R (eds) Movement, stability and low back pain. Churchill Livingstone, Edinburgh, ch 19, p 235

Grieve G P 1981 Common vertebral joint problems. Churchill Livingstone, Edinburgh

Grieve G P 1981 The hip. Physiotherapy 69: 196

Grieve G P (ed) 1986 Modern manual therapy of the vertebral column. Churchill Livingstone, Edinburgh

Grob K R, Neuhuber W L, Kissling R O 1995 Innervation of the sacroiliac joint of the human. Zeitschrift für Rheumatologie 54: 117–122

Hagen R 1974 Pelvic girdle relaxation from an orthopaedic point of view. Acta Orthopaedica Scandinavica 45: 550

Hanson P, Sonesson B 1994 The anatomy of the iliolumbar ligament. Archives of Physical Medicine and Rehabilitation 75: 1245–1246

Hartman L 1997 Handbook of osteopathic technique, 3rd edn. Chapman & Hall, London

Heiberg E, Aarseth S P 1997 Epidemiology of pelvic pain and low back pain in pregnant women. In: Vleeming A, Mooney V, Dorman T, Snijders C, Stoeckart R (eds) Movement, stability and low back pain. Churchill Livingstone, Edinburgh, ch 32, p 405

Herzog W, Read L, Conway P J W, Shaw L D, McEwen M C 1989 Reliability of motion palpation procedures to detect sacroiliac joint fixations. Journal of Manipulative Physical Therapy 12(2): 86–92

Hesch J 1997 Evaluation and treatment of the most common patterns of sacroiliac joint dysfunction. In: Vleeming A, Mooney V, Dorman T, Snijders C, Stoeckart R (eds) Movement, stability and low back pain. Churchill Livingstone, Edinburgh, ch 42, p 535

Hesch J, Aisenbrey J, Guarino J 1992 Manual therapy evaluation of the pelvic joints using palpatory and articular spring tests. In: Vleeming A, Mooney V, Snijders C J, Dorman T (eds) First interdisciplinary world congress on low back pain and its relation to the sacroiliac joint. San Diego, CA, 5–6 November, p 435

Hides J A, Stokes M J, Saide M, Jull G A, Cooper D H 1994 Evidence of lumbar multifidus muscles wasting ipsilateral to symptoms in patients with acute/subacute low back pain. Spine 19(2): 165–177

Hides J A, Richardson C A, Jull G A 1996 Multifidus recovery is not automatic following resolution of acute first episode low back pain. Spine 21(23): 2763–2769

Hodges P W 1997c New advances in exercise to rehabilitate spinal stabilization, course notes, Delta Orthopaedic Physiotherapy Clinic, Delta, B.C., Canada, December 6, 7, 1997

Hodges P W, Richardson C A 1996 Inefficient muscular stabilization of the lumbar spine associated with low back pain. A motor control evaluation of transversus abdominis. Spine 21(22): 2640–2650

Hodges P W, Richardson C A 1997a Contraction of the abdominal muscles associated with movement of the lower limb. Physical Therapy 77: 132–144

Hodges P W, Richardson C A 1997b Feedforward contraction of transversus abdominis is not affected by the direction of arm movement. Experimental Brain Research 114: 362–370

Inman V T, Ralston H J, Todd F 1981 Human walking. Williams & Wilkins, Baltimore

Irion J M, 1992 Use of the gym ball in rehabilitation of spinal dysfunction. Orthopaedic Physical Therapy Clinics of North America—Exercise Technologies 1(2): 375–398

Jacob H A C, Kissling R O 1995 The mobility of the sacroiliac joints in healthy volunteers between 20 and 50 years of age. Clinical Biomechanics 10(7): 352–361

Janda V 1986 Muscle weakness and inhibition (pseudoparesis) in back pain syndromes. In: Grieve G P (ed) Modern manual therapy of the vertebral column. Churchill Livingstone, Edinburgh, ch 19, p 197

Janda V 1978 Muscles, central nervous motor regulation and back problems. In: Korr I (ed) The neurobiologic mechanisms in manipulative therapy. Plenum Press, London, p 27

Jarcho J 1929 Value of Walcher position in contracted pelvis with special reference to its effect on true conjugate diameter. Surgery, Gynecology and Obstetrics 49: 854

Jull G A, Bogduk N, Marsland A 1988 The accuracy of manual diagnosis for cervical zygapophyseal joint pain syndromes. Medical Journal of Australia 148: 233–236

Kapandji I A 1970 The physiology of the joints II: the lower limb, 2nd edn. Churchill Livingstone, Edinburgh

Kapandji I A 1974 The physiology of the joints III: the trunk and vertebral column, 2nd edn. Churchill Livingstone, Edinburgh

Kappel D A, Zilber S, Ketchum L D 1973 In vivo electrophysiology of tendons and applied current during tendon healing. In: Llaurado J G, Battocletti J H (eds) Biologic and clinical effects of low-frequency magnetic and electric fields. C C Thomas, Illinois, ch 21, p 252

Kappler R E 1982 Postural balance and motion patterns. Journal of the American Osteopathic Association 81(9): 598

Keagy R D, Brumlik J 1966 Direct electromyography of the psoas major muscle in man. Journal of Bone and Joint Surgery 48A: 1377

Kendall F P, Kendall McCreary E, Provance P G 1993 Muscles testing and function, 4th edn. Williams & Wilkins, Baltimore

Kirkaldy-Willis W H (ed) 1983 Managing low back pain. Churchill Livingstone, New York

Kirkaldy-Willis W H, Hill R J 1979 A more precise diagnosis for low back pain. Spine 4: 102

Kirkaldy-Willis W H, Wedge J H, Yong-Hing K, Reilly J 1978 Pathology and pathogenesis of lumbar spondylosis and stenosis. Spine 3: 319

Kissling R O, Jacob H A C 1997 The mobility of sacroiliac joints in healthy subjects. In: Vleeming A, Mooney V, Dorman T, Snijders C, Stoeckart R (eds) Movement, stability and low back pain. Churchill Livingstone, Edinburgh, ch 12, p 177

Kristiansson P 1997 S-Relaxin and pelvic pain in pregnant women. In: Vleeming A, Mooney V, Dorman T, Snijders C, Stoeckart R (eds) Movement, stability and low back pain. Churchill Livingstone, Edinburgh, ch 34, p 421

Laslett M 1997 Pain provocation sacroiliac joint tests: reliability and prevalence. In: Vleeming A, Mooney V, Dorman T, Snijders C, Stoeckart R (eds) Movement, stability and low back pain. Churchill Livingstone, Edinburgh, ch 23, p 287

Laslett M, Williams W 1994 The reliability of selected pain provocation tests for sacroiliac joint pathology. Spine 19(11): 1243–1249

Lavignolle B, Vital J M, Senegas J, Destandau J, Toson B, Bouyx P, Morlier P, Delorme G, Calabet A 1983 An approach to the functional anatomy of the sacroiliac joints in vivo. Anatomica Clinica 5: 169–176

Lawson T L, Foley W D, Carrera G F, Berland L L 1982 The sacroiliac joints: anatomic, plain roentgenographic, and computed tomographic analysis. Journal of Computer Assisted Tomography 6(2): 307

Lee D G 1989 The pelvic girdle. Churchill Livingstone, Edinburgh

Lee D G 1992 Intra-articular versus extra-articular dysfunction of the sacroiliac joint—a method of differentiation. IFOMT Proceedings, 5th international conference. Vail, Colorado, p 69–71

Lee D G 1997a Instability of the sacroiliac joint and the consequences for gait. In: Vleeming A, Mooney V, Dorman T, Snijders C, Stoeckart R (eds) Movement, stability and low back pain. Churchill Livingstone, Edinburgh, ch 18, p 231

Lee D G 1997b Treatment of pelvic instability. In: Vleeming A, Mooney V, Dorman T, Snijders C, Stoeckart R (eds) Movement, stability and low back pain. Churchill Livingstone, Edinburgh, ch 37, 445

Lee D G, Walsh M C 1996 A workbook of manual therapy techniques for the vertebral column and pelvic girdle, 2nd edn. Nascent, Vancouver

Levin S M 1997 A different approach to the mechanics of the human pelvis: tensegrity. In: Vleeming A, Mooney V, Dorman T, Snijders C, Stoeckart R (eds) Movement, stability and low back pain. Churchill Livingstone, Edinburgh, ch 10 p 157

Lovett R W 1903 A contribution to the study of the mechanics of the spine. American Journal of Anatomy 2: 457

Luk K D K, Ho H C, Leong J C Y 1986 The iliolumbar ligament: a study of its anatomy, development and clinical significance. Journal of Bone and Joint Surgery 68B: 197

Lynch F W 1920 The pelvic articulations during pregnancy, labor, and the puerperium. Surgery, Gynecology and Obstetrics 30: 575

MacConaill M A, Basmajian J V 1977 Muscles and movements; a basis for human kinesiology, 2nd edn. Krieger, New York

MacDonald G R, Hunt T E 1951 Sacro-iliac joint observations on the gross and histological changes in the various age groups. Canadian Medical Association Journal 66: 157

MacNab I 1977 Backache. Williams & Wilkins, Baltimore

Maigne J Y 1997 Lateral dynamic X-rays in the sitting position and coccygeal discography in common coccydynia. In: Vleeming A, Mooney V, Dorman T, Snijders C, Stoeckart R (eds) Movement, stability and low back pain. Churchill Livingstone, Edinburgh, ch 30, p 385

Maigne J Y, Aivaliklis A, Pfefer F 1996 Results of sacroiliac joint double block and value of sacroiliac pain provocation tests in 54 patients with low back pain. Spine 21: 1889–1892

Maxwell T D 1978 The piriformis muscle and its relation to the long-legged syndrome. Journal of the Canadian Chiropractic Association July: 51

McNeill Alexander R 1995 Elasticity in mammalian backs. In: Vleeming A, Mooney V, Dorman T, Snijders C (eds) Second interdisciplinary world congress on low back pain: The integrated function of the lumbar spine and sacroiliac joint, Part 1, San Diego, CA, 9–11 November, p 7

McNeill Alexander R 1997 Elasticity in human and animal backs. In: Vleeming A, Mooney V, Dorman T, Snijders C, Stoeckart R (eds) Movement, stability and low back pain. Churchill Livingstone, Edinburgh, ch 17 p 227

McQueen P M 1977 The piriformis syndrome. Physiotherapy Society Manipulation Newsletter, Melbourne 8: 1

Meisenbach R O 1911 Sacro-iliac relaxation; with analysis of eighty-four cases. Surgery, Gynecology and Obstetrics 12: 411

Melzak R, Wall P D 1965 Pain mechanisms: a new theory. Science 150: 971

Mennell J B 1952 The science and art of joint manipulation. Churchill, London

Mens J M A, Vleeming A, Stoeckart R, Stam J H, Snijders C J 1996 Understanding peripartum pelvic pain: implications of a patient survey. Spine 21(11): 1303–1369

Mens J M A, Vleeming A, Snijders C J, Stam H J 1997 Active straight leg raising test: a clinical approach to the load transfer function of the pelvic girdle. In: Vleeming A, Mooney V, Dorman T, Snijders C, Stoeckart R (eds) Movement, stability and low back pain. Churchill Livingstone, Edinburgh, ch 35, p 425

Mester E 1971 Effects of laser rays on wound healing. American Journal of Surgery 122: 532

Meyer G H 1878 Der Mechanismus der Symphysis sacroiliaca. Archiv für Anatomie und Physiologie 1: 1

Miller J A A, Schultz A B, Andersson G B J 1987 Load-displacement behavior of sacro-iliac joints. Journal of Orthopedic Research 5: 92–101

Mitchell F 1965 Structural pelvic function. Year Book: Academy of Applied Osteopathy. Carmel, California

Mixter W J, Barr J S 1934 Rupture of intervertebral disc with involvement of the spinal cord. New England Journal of Medicine 211: 210

Mooney V, 1997 Sacroiliac joint dysfunction. In: Vleeming A, Mooney V, Dorman T, Snijders C, Stoeckart R (eds) Movement, stability and low back pain. Churchill Livingstone, Edinburgh, ch 2, p 37

Nelson H, Jurmain R 1985 Introduction to physical anthropology, 3rd edn. West Publishing, St Paul

Ostgaard H C 1997 Lumbar back and posterior pelvic pain in pregnancy. In: Vleeming A, Mooney V, Dorman T, Snijders C, Stoeckart R (eds) Movement, stability and low back pain. Churchill Livingstone, Edinburgh, ch 33, p 411

Panjabi M M 1992 The stabilizing system of the spine. I: Function, dysfunction, adaptation, and enhancement. Journal of Spinal Disorders 5(4): 383–389

Paydar D, Thiel H, Gemmell H 1994 Intra- and interexaminer reliability of certain pelvic palpatory procedures and the sitting flexion test for sacroiliac joint mobility and dysfunction. Journal of Neuromusculoskeletal Medicine 2(2) 65–69

Peacock E E 1984 Wound repair, 3rd edn. W B Saunders, London

Pearcy M, Tibrewal S B 1984 Axial rotation and lateral bending in the normal lumbar spine measured by three-dimensional radiography. Spine 9: 582

Pitkin H C, Pheasant H C 1936 Sacroarthrogenetic telalagia II. A study of sacral mobility. Journal of Bone and Joint Surgery 18: 365

Potter N A, Rothstein J 1985 Intertester reliability for selected clinical tests of the sacroiliac joint. Physical Therapy 65(11): 1671–1675

Reid D C 1992 Sports injury assessment and rehabilitation. Churchill Livingstone, New York

Reilly J, Yong-Hing K, MacKay R W, Kirkaldy-Willis W H 1978 Pathological anatomy of the lumbar spine. In: Helfet A J, Gruebel-Lee D M (eds) Disorders of the lumbar spine. J B Lippincott, Philadelphia

Resnick D, Niwayama G, Goergen T G 1975 Degenerative disease of the sacroiliac joint. Journal of Investigative Radiology 10: 608

Richardson C A, Jull G A 1994 Concepts of assessment and rehabilitation for active lumbar stability. In: Boyling J D, Palastanga N (eds) Grieve's modern manual therapy of the vertebral column, 2nd edn. Churchill Livingstone, Edinburgh, p 705

Richardson C A, Jull G A 1995 Muscle control—pain control. What exercises would you prescribe? Manual Therapy 1: 2–10

Richardson C A, Jull G A, Hodges P W, Hides J A 1996 New advances in exercise to rehabilitate spinal stabilization, course notes, Delta Orthopaedic Physiotherapy Clinic, Delta, B.C., Canada, November 12, 13, 1996

Rizk N N 1980 A new description of the anterior abdominal wall in man and mammals. Journal of Anatomy 131: 373–385

Rodman P S, McHenry M 1980 Bioenergetics and the origin of hominid bipedalism. American Journal of Physical Anthropology 52: 103

Rohen J W, Yokochi C 1983 Color atlas of anatomy, a photographic study of the human body. F K Schattauer, Stuttgart, and Igaku-Shoin, Tokyo

Romer A S 1959 A shorter version of the vertebrate body. W B Saunders, Philadelphia

Rothman R H, Simeone F A 1975 Spine, Vol. IV. W B Saunders, London

Rowinski M J 1985 Afferent neurobiology of the joint. In: Gould J A, Davies J D (eds) Orthopaedic and sports physical therapy. C V Mosby, St. Louis, p 50–63

Sapsford R R, Hodges P W, Richardson C A 1998 Activation of the abdominal muscles is a normal response to contraction of the pelvic floor. Submitted

Sashin D 1930 A critical analysis of the anatomy and the pathologic changes of the sacro-iliac joints. Journal of Bone and Joint Surgery 12: 891

Schunke G B 1938 The anatomy and development of the sacro-iliac joint in man. The Anatomical Record 72: 313

Schwarzer A C, Aprill C N, Bogduk N 1995 The sacroiliac joint in chronic low back pain. Spine 20: 31–37

Siffert R S, Feldman D J 1980 The growing hip. Acta Orthopaedica Belgica 46: 443

Singleton M C, LeVeau B F 1975 The hip joint: structure, stability, and stress. Physical Therapy 55: 957

Smidt G L 1995 Sacroiliac kinematics for reciprocal straddle positions. In: Vleeming A, Mooney V, Dorman T, Snijders C (eds) Second interdisciplinary world congress on low back pain: the integrated function of the lumbar spine and sacroiliac joint, Part 2, San Diego, CA, 9–11, November, p 695

Snijders C J, Vleeming A, Stoeckart R 1993a Transfer of lumbosacral load to iliac bones and legs. 1: Biomechanics of self-bracing of the sacroiliac joints and its significance for treatment and exercise. Clinical biomechanics 8: 285–294

Snijders C J, Vleeming A, Stoeckart R 1993b Transfer of lumbosacral load to iliac bones and legs. 2: Loading of the sacroiliac joints when lifting in a stooped posture. Clinical biomechanics 8: 295–301

Snijders C J, Slagter A H E, Strik R van, Vleeming A, Stoeckart R, Stam H J 1995 Why leg-crossing? The influence of common postures on abdominal muscle activity. Spine 20(18): 1989–1993

Snijders C J, Vleeming A, Stoeckart R, Mens J M A, Kleinrensink G J 1997 Biomechanics of the interface between spine and pelvis in different postures. In: Vleeming A, Mooney V, Dorman T, Snijders C, Stoeckart R (eds) Movement, stability and low back pain. Churchill Livingstone, Edinburgh, ch 6, p 103

Solonen K A 1957 The sacro-iliac joint in the light of anatomical roentgenological and clinical studies. Acta Orthopaedica Scandinavica Suppl 26

Stark S D 1997 The stark reality of stretching. Peanut Butter, Vancouver

Stein P L, Rowe B M 1982 Physical anthropology, 3rd edn. McGraw-Hill, New York

Stokes I A F 1986 Three-dimensional biplanar radiography of the lumbar spine. In: Grieve G P (ed) Modern manual therapy of the vertebral column. Churchill Livingstone, Edinburgh, ch 54, p 576

Strayer L M 1971 Embryology of the human hip joint. Clinical Orthopaedics 74: 221

Sturesson B 1997 Movement of the sacroiliac joint: a fresh look. In: Vleeming A, Mooney V, Dorman T, Snijders C, Stoeckart R (eds) Movement, stability and l ow back pain. Churchill Livingstone, Edinburgh, ch 11, p 171

Sturesson B, Selvik G, Uden A 1989 Movements of the sacroiliac joints: a roentgen stereophotogrammetric analysis. Spine 14 (2): 162–165

Sunderland S 1978 Traumatized nerves, roots and ganglia: musculo-skeletal factors and neuropathological consequences. In: Korr (ed) The neurobiologic mechanisms in manipulative therapy. Plenum Press, London, p 137

Swindler D R, Wood C D 1982 An atlas of primate gross anatomy: baboon, chimpanzee, and man. Robert E Krieger, Florida

Taylor J R, Twomey L T 1986 Age changes in lumbar zygapophyseal joints: observations on structure and function. Spine 11(7): 739–744

Taylor J T, Twomey L T 1992 Structure and function of lumbar zygapophyseal (facet) joints: a review. Journal of Orthopaedic Medicine 14(3): 71–78

Taylor J T, Twomey L T, Corker M 1990 Bone and soft tissue injuries in post-mortem lumbar spines. Paraplegia 28: 119–129

Travell J G, Rinzler S H 1952 The myofascial genesis of pain. Postgraduate Medicine 11: 425

Trotter M 1937 Accessory sacro-iliac articulations. American Journal of Physical Anthropology 22: 247

Tuttle R H (ed) 1975 Primate functional morphology. Mouton, The Hague

Twomey L T, Taylor J R 1985 A quantitative study of the role of the posterior vertebral elements in sagittal movements of the lumbar vertebral column. In: Glasgow E F, Twomey L T, Scull E R, Kleynhans A M (eds) Aspects of manipulative therapy, 2nd edn. Churchill Livingstone, Melbourne, ch 4, p 34

Twomey L T, Taylor J R 1986 The effects of aging on the lumbar intervertebral discs. In: Grieve G P (ed) Modern manual therapy of the vertebral column. Churchill Livingstone, Edinburgh, ch 12, p 129

Twomey L T, Taylor J R, Taylor M M 1989 Unsuspected damage to lumbar zygapophyseal (facet) joints after motor-vehicle accidents. Medical Journal of Australia 151: 210–217

Uhtoff H K 1993 Prenatal development of the iliolumbar ligament. Journal of Bone and Joint Surgery (Britain) 75: 93–95

Vicenzino G, Twomey L 1993 Sideflexion induced lumbar spine conjunct rotation and its influencing factors. Australian Physiotherapy 39(4): 299–306

Vlaeyen J W S, Kole-Snijders A M J, Heuts P H T G, van Eek H 1997 Behavioral analysis, fear of movement/(re)injury and behavioral rehabilitation in chronic low back pain. In: Vleeming A, Mooney V, Dorman T, Snijders C, Stoeckart R (eds) Movement, stability and low back pain. Churchill Livingstone, Edinburgh, ch 36, p 435

Vleeming A, Stoeckart R, Snijders C J 1989a The sacrotuberous ligament: a conceptual approach to its dynamic role in stabilizing the sacroiliac joint. Clinical Biomechanics 4: 201–203

Vleeming A, Wingerden J P van, Snijders C J, Stoeckart R, Stijnen T 1989b Load application to the sacrotuberous ligament: influences on sacroiliac joint mechanics. Clinical Biomechanics 4: 204–209

Vleeming A, Stoeckart R, Volkers A C W, Snijders C J 1990a Relation between form and function in the sacroiliac joint. 1: Clinical anatomical aspects. Spine 15(2): 130–132

Vleeming A, Volkers A C W, Snijders C J, Stoeckart R 1990b Relation between form and function in the sacroiliac joint. 2: Biomechanical aspects. Spine 15(2): 133–136

Vleeming A, Mooney V, Snijders C, Dorman T (eds) 1992a First interdisciplinary world congress on low back pain and its relation to the sacroiliac joint, San Diego, CA, 5–6 November

Vleeming A, Wingerden J P van, Dijkstra P F, Stoeckart R, Snijders C J, Stijnen T 1992b Mobility in the SI-joints in old people: a kinematic and radiologic study. Clinical Biomechanics 7: 170–176

Vleeming A, Pool-Goudzwaard A L, Stoeckart R, Wingerden J P van, Snijders C J 1995a The posterior layer of the thoracolumbar fascia: its function in load transfer from spine to legs. Spine 20: 753–758

Vleeming A, Mooney V, Dorman T, Snijders C (eds) 1995b Second interdisciplinary world congress on low back pain: The integrated function of the lumbar spine and sacroiliac joint, Part 1 & 2, San Diego, CA, 9–11 November

Vleeming A, Pool-Goudzwaard A L, Hammudoghlu D, Stoeckart R, Snijders C J, Mens J M A 1996 The function of the long dorsal sacroiliac ligament: its implication for understanding low back pain. Spine 21(5): 556–562

Vleeming A, Snijders C J, Stoeckart R, Mens J M A 1997 The role of the sacroiliac joints in coupling between spine, pelvis, legs and arms. In: Vleeming A, Mooney V, Dorman T, Snijders C, Stoeckart R (eds) Movement, stability and low back pain. Churchill Livingstone, Edinburgh, ch 3 p 53

Walheim G G, Selvik G 1984 Mobility of the pubic symphysis. Clinical Orthopaedics and Related Research 191: 129–135

Walker J M 1980a Morphological variants in the human fetal hip joint. Journal of Bone and Joint Surgery 62A: 1073

Walker J M 1980b Growth characteristics of the fetal ligament of the head of femur: significance in congenital hip disease. Yale Journal of Biology and Medicine 53: 307

Walker J M 1981 Histological study of the fetal development of the human acetabulum and labrum: significance in congenital hip disease. Yale Journal of Biology and Medicine 54: 255

Walker J M 1984 Age changes in the sacroiliac joint. Proceedings of the International Federation of Orthopaedic Manipulative Therapists—5th, Vancouver, p 250

Walker J M 1986 Age-related differences in the human sacroiliac joint: a histological study; implications for therapy. Journal of Orthopaedic and Sports Physical Therapy 7: 325

Warwick R, Williams P (eds) 1989 Gray's anatomy, 37th edn. Longman, London

Watanabe R S 1974 Embryology of the human hip. Clinical Orthopaedics 98: 8

Webster D F, Harvey W, Dyson M, Pond J B 1980 The role of ultrasound-induced cavitation in the 'in vitro' stimulation of collagen synthesis in human fibroblasts. Ultrasonic 18: 33

Weisl H 1954 The articular surfaces of the sacro-iliac joint and their relation to the movements of the sacrum. Acta Anatomica 22: 1

Weisl H 1955 The movements of the sacro-iliac joint. Acta Anatomica 23: 80

White A A, Panjabi M M 1978 The basic kinematics of the human spine. Spine 3: 12

White S G, Sahrmann S A 1994 A movement system balance approach to management of musculoskeletal pain. In: Grant R (ed) Physical therapy of the cervical and thoracic spine, 2nd edn. Churchill Livingstone, New York

Wilder D G, Pope M H, Frymoyer J W 1980 The functional topography of the sacroiliac joint. Spine 5: 575

Willard F H 1997 The muscular, ligamentous and neural structure of the low back and its relation to back pain. In: Vleeming A, Mooney V, Dorman T, Snijders C, Stoeckart R (eds) Movement, stability and low back pain. Churchill Livingstone, Edinburgh, ch 1 p 3

Williams P E, Goldspink G 1978 Changes in sarcomere length and physiological properties in immobilised muscle. Journal of Anatomy 127: 459

Wingerden J P van, Vleeming A, Snijders C J, Stoeckart R 1993 A functional-anatomical approach to the spine-pelvis mechanism: interaction between the biceps femoris muscle and the sacrotuberous ligament. European Spine Journal 2: 140–144

Wroblewski B M 1978 Pain in osteoarthrosis of the hip. Practitioner: 1315: 140

Wyke B D 1981 The neurology of joints: a review of general principles. Clinics in Rheumatic Diseases 7: 223

Wyke B D 1985 Articular neurology and manipulative therapy. In: Glasgow E F, Twomey L T, Scull E R, Kleynhans A M (eds) Aspects of manipulative therapy, 2nd edn. Churchill Livingstone, Melbourne, ch 11, p 72

Young J 1940 Relaxation of the pelvic joints in pregnancy: pelvic arthropathy of pregnancy. Journal of Obstetrics and Gynecology 47: 493

Young J Z 1981 The life of vertebrates, 3rd edn. Clarendon Press, Oxford

Index

There are three videos linked to this book:

Examination of the Articular Function of the Pelvic Girdle
This reviews five key tests for determining the ability of the pelvis to transfer load from the trunk to the lower extremity.

Manual Therapy Techniques for the Sacroiliac Joint
This demonstrates the mobilization (active and passive) and manipulation techniques used to restore function to the sacroiliac joint.

Exercises for the Unstable Pelvis
This describes the principles upon which this evidence-based exercise program is based, and demonstrates the progression of exercises used for patients with impaired load transfer through the pelvic girdle.

Further information can be obtained from:

Delta Orthopaedic Physiotherapy clinic
302 11950 80th Avenue
Delta, B.C.
Canada
V4C 1Y2

Fax: 604 591-3660 or email: dopc@direct.ca